"The authors have done a masterful job describing how we can use language towards ourselves and others more mindfully to support a healthy self-image that can lead us to live more authentic lives."

—Staffan Elgelid, PhD, PT, GCFP, C-IAYT, RYT 500, coauthor of
Yoga Therapy for Stress & Anxiety and *Yoga Therapy:
A Personalized Approach for Your Active Lifestyle*

"Butera and Kreatsoulas have created a pragmatic, holistic, and thoughtful approach to finding peace and friendship with one's body. Your body holds a wisdom and a language of its own. *Body Mindful Yoga* helps you connect to that wisdom while simultaneously increasing your understanding of the messages your body sends you through a lens of compassion, clarity, and confidence. A must-read."

—Lisa Diers, RDN, LD, E-RYT, yoga therapist and founder of
Yoga and Nutrition Consulting, LLC

"Jennifer and Robert help us examine and befriend the parts of us that are silent, loud, unmet, or unrequited. This book empowers anyone to build a conscientious bridge to escort their inner worth towards stronger and brighter social bonds....*Body Mindful Yoga* unlaces the complexity of under-examined self-dialogue and engages the unspoken sentiments of heart, soul, and mind so that they are no longer invisible. This helpful book is a gift to movement instructors, mental health professionals, teachers, and anyone seeking to enrich their relationship with self and body."

—Jill Miller, author of *The Roll Model* and creator of Yoga Tune Up

"*Body Mindful Yoga* offers a fresh and important perspective with depth and clarity. Liberate yourself and claim your full potential with this stellar method of making friends with your body. This self-loving study of your body's story opens doors to confidence, compassion, insight, and personal/societal evolution. I highly recommend this book for yoga teachers and therapists, health professionals, and anyone who wishes to discover more about having a nurturing relationship with the body. The exploratory exercises and concrete steps support you in learning to listen to your authentic voice and affirm the truth of the body you're in!"

—Erin Byron, registered psychotherapist and
author of *Yoga for the Creative Soul*

"*Body Mindful Yoga* offers many insights into the body image crisis that our culture is currently experiencing. Through meaningful examination and powerful reflective practices, readers are guided to deconstruct deep-seated body image beliefs and transform them into positive and uplifting new paradigms. Guidance is offered for integrating new dialogues, and the tone of the book is one of personal empowerment and potential for social change. I highly recommend this book."

—Kristen Butera, E-RYT 500, C-IAYT, author of *Yoga Therapy:*
A Personalized Approach for Your Active Lifestyle

body
mindful
yoga

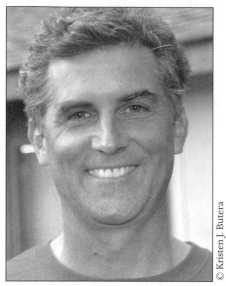

Robert Butera, PhD

Robert Butera, MDiv, PhD (Devon, PA), founded YogaLife Institute in Pennsylvania, where he trains yoga teachers and Comprehensive Yoga Therapists. Robert's PhD at CA Institute of Integral Studies focused on Yoga Therapy. He authored *The Pure Heart of Yoga*, *Meditation for Your Life*, and *Yoga Therapy for Stress & Anxiety*. Visit him at www.YogaLifeInstitute.com.

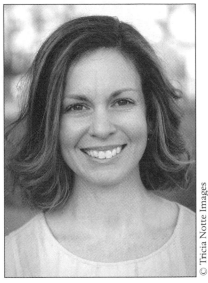

© Tricia Notte Images

Jennifer Kreatsoulas, PhD

Jennifer Kreatsoulas, PhD (Collegeville, PA), is a certified yoga therapist and inspirational speaker. She presents, writes, and leads workshops, trainings, and retreats on eating disorder recovery and body image. She also provides yoga therapy via phone or online and from YogaLife Institute in Wayne, PA. Visit her at www.yoga4eatingdisorders.com.

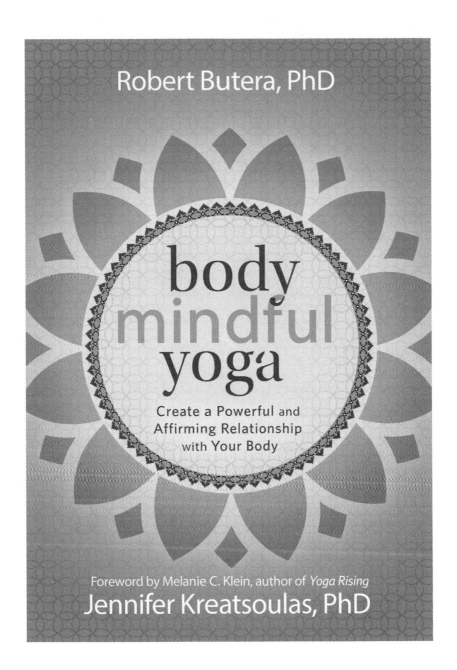

Robert Butera, PhD

body
mindful
yoga

Create a Powerful and
Affirming Relationship
with Your Body

Foreword by Melanie C. Klein, author of *Yoga Rising*

Jennifer Kreatsoulas, PhD

Llewellyn Publications
Woodbury, Minnesota

FIRST EDITION
First Printing, 2018

Cover design by Shira Atakpu
Interior illustrations by Mary Ann Zapalac

Llewellyn Publications is a registered trademark of Llewellyn Worldwide Ltd.

Library of Congress Cataloging-in-Publication Data
Names: Butera, Robert, author.
Title: Body mindful yoga : create a powerful and affirming relationship with
   your body / by Robert Butera, PhD, and Jennifer Kreatsoulas, PhD.
Description: First Edition. | Woodbury : Llewellyn Worldwide, Ltd., 2018. |
   Includes index.
Identifiers: LCCN 2018029960 (print) | LCCN 2018041234 (ebook) | ISBN
   9780738756936 (ebook) | ISBN 9780738756738 (alk. paper)
Subjects: LCSH: Yoga. | Body image. | Mindfulness (Psychology)
Classification: LCC BF697.5.B63 (ebook) | LCC BF697.5.B63 B88 2018 (print) |
   DDC 613.7/046—dc23
LC record available at https://lccn.loc.gov/2018029960

Llewellyn Publications
A Division of Llewellyn Worldwide Ltd.
2143 Wooddale Drive
Woodbury, MN 55125-2989
www.llewellyn.com

Printed in the United States of America

Other Books by Robert Butera, PhD

Llewellyn's Complete Book of Mindful Living (with Erin Byron, MA)
(Llewellyn, 2016)

Yoga Therapy for Stress & Anxiety (with Erin Byron, MA)
(Llewellyn, 2015)

Meditation for Your Life
(Llewellyn, 2012)

The Pure Heart of Yoga
(Llewellyn, 2009)

To our readers and future generations,
may your words affirm your body and embrace your wisdom.

Contents

Step 3: Love

Chapter 11:
Body Mindful Practices for Your Inner Life ... 147

Step 4: Live

Chapter 12:
How to Be a Body Mindful Ambassador ... 179

Exercises

Chapter 11

Chapter 12

Yoga Poses

Disclaimer

The practices, movements, and methods described in this book should not be used as an alternative to professional diagnosis or treatment. The authors and publisher of this book are not responsible in any manner whatsoever for any injury or negative effects that might occur through following the instructions and advice contained in this book. Before beginning any treatment or exercise program, it is recommended that you consult medical professionals to determine whether you should undertake this course of practice.

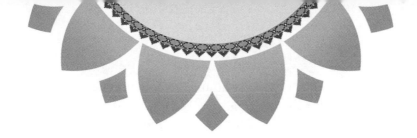

Foreword

Language, the symbol systems we use to communicate both verbally and nonverbally, is the foundation of our cultural reality. Without language, culture would not exist. It is language that allows us to have a shared reality. The words we use to communicate, the ways in which we communicate, and the words and meanings we have yet to create are the seeds of change. Oftentimes, social change is imagined in terms of large-scale events, while the power of smaller-level actions, like shifting our language, is undervalued or overlooked entirely.

Can we become more aware of how we communicate and evaluate ourselves and others? Can we become conscious of the ways in which the larger sociopolitical landscape informs both and leads to measures of worth and value? Can we begin to track these patterns and then choose to create a shift? Absolutely! Yoga and mindfulness tools elevate our consciousness and attune us to the often taken-for-granted aspects of our cultural narrative and, specifically, our internal dialogue, which is an essential component and contribution to the larger cultural messages around body acceptance and peace. In fact, this is where yoga and mindfulness tools become essential, as *Body Mindful Yoga* so poignantly makes clear and relevant. If body acceptance and peace are the desired outcome, we must become conscious of the larger cultural narrative and our own internal dialogue. Yoga and mindfulness tools provide us with the opportunity to become attuned to both the cultural narratives and our personal stories. And when we become aware, we create opportunities to make new choices that empower rather than undermine our sense of self and our relationship with our bodies.

The task of deconstructing and recreating our framework of understanding can seem daunting. How do I begin? What guide is available? What tools can I harness? Well, guess what? You're holding that powerful tool in your hands right now. Loaded with insight, wisdom, and practical tools and mindfulness practices, *Body Mindful Yoga* offers a clear path to change the ways we think and feel about ourselves and others for all who read it and take action. This book is a guide you can refer to over and over again as you take your personal insight and experience off the yoga mat (or the meditation cushion) and out into the world, because a shift in perspective and, most importantly, a shift in *being* requires all of us to step into our power and role-model how to become agents of change in whatever way is most authentic to us. And it begins with our words. This book will undoubtedly support you on that path.

I'm passionate about the messages and ideas *Body Mindful Yoga* teaches, because I'm also on a mission to radically alter the way we see and value ourselves as well as the way we view, evaluate, and relate to others and the world at large. This mission is the root of a movement that continues to grow and reach into all areas of our lives, especially our hearts, minds, and spirits. I invite you to dive into the beauty and wisdom of this book with the clear understanding that it is a gift to our individual and collective liberation from the ways in which we limit our full potential and keep ourselves small and our voices muffled. *Body Mindful Yoga* is one step in a longer ongoing journey leading you and the world to self-acceptance and, possibly, full-blown radical self-love.

When we come to a place of self-acceptance and peace, we inevitably radiate that energy into every corner of our lives. When we end the war on ourselves and our bodies, we become beacons of light for others and we amplify the frequency of the collective. Our personal liberation is tied to the collective liberation of *every* body, regardless of size, age, race or ethnicity, gender identity or sexual orientation, class, dis/ability, nationality, or religious affiliation.

Body Mindful Yoga is part of a movement rooted in social justice and anti-oppression. This movement recognizes that the personal is political, that our individual lives and experiences are directly tied to the structures and systems of the cultures we reside in, cultures we create and recreate with every interaction. It is a grassroots movement in all its messy, beautiful, and creative glory. It is a movement full of heart and fueled by an unwavering love for ourselves, each other, the world we inhabit, and the possibilities of humanity. When we can reframe our perspective, we shift our reality. When we consciously integrate and wield language that shifts the framework of our individual reality, we create shifts in the collective consciousness. In this way, we turn the tide of the dominant culture with our words. *Body Mindful Yoga* provides insight and tools for taking personal action toward manifesting this kind of powerful shift.

As a sociologist, I emphasize the ability of our cultural landscape's ability to be changed. I share this message with my students and encourage them to investigate, challenge, and reconstruct their personal and our collective cultural framework. We take for granted not only the ways in which society and the cultural fabric informs our development of self and the lens through which we view the world, but also the ways in which we have the power to create change. My students find it liberating to know that they do not need to accept things as they are. Through this book, I invite you to embrace the possibilities of change and investigate your deeply held ideals and assumptions. It can feel a little uncomfortable at times, but that is quickly outweighed by the scope of boundless opportunities for creating an affirming, empowering, and accepting relationship with yourself and your body.

Never underestimate the power of the words we choose and use. We wield power. Let's choose our words consciously and wisely. Let's wield our words as swords of light and good.

Here's to our individual and collective liberation!

Melanie C. Klein
Santa Monica, CA
November 2017

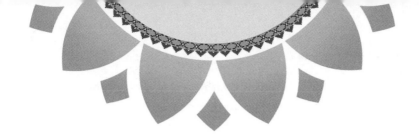

Introduction

This book is an invitation to participate in a story that belongs to you and only you. It is the story of your relationship with your body. That statement may sound odd, since we typically think of the stories we tell from our lives to be about things like where we grew up or went to school, the sports we played or hobbies we enjoyed, how we met our significant other, or milestone events. Our stories might also be about travels, aspirations, illness, pain, and loss. These are the stories we tell at dinner with friends, holiday gatherings with family, and other social events with peers, colleagues, and acquaintances.

Just as valid as the stories we share about our accomplishments and pursuits are the narratives that show up every day in our self-talk and exchanges with others about our bodies. Our perceptions and beliefs about how we look, should look, or want to look can occupy a significant portion of our inner dialogue and sway how we see ourselves in the world without us even realizing it. Be it confident, strong, accepting, unhappy, embarrassed, or ashamed, the way we feel about our bodies in any given moment is expressed through our words (including what is *not* being said), actions, and physical demeanor in our daily conversations with ourselves and others.

Social norms have made it acceptable to openly and frequently express dissatisfaction with our physical appearance. Conversely, conveying a sense of pride or contentment with our bodies runs the risk of being interpreted as self-centered or even narcissistic. Mixed messages such as these may leave the impression that our bodies are a problem, and we may innocently fall into the pattern of talking disparagingly about our bodies or purposely refraining from showing appreciation or admiration for our bodies' abilities and attributes. Ultimately, these ways of relating to our bodies can keep us stuck in stories that focus on discontent with our physical appearance.

Relating to our bodies in a caring or thoughtful way as we would with a close friend is an uncommon notion in our society. We are much more familiar with the concepts of fixing, changing, taming, control-ling, or improving our bodies than validating, affirming, or honoring them. Combative words such as these permeate the social conscious-ness, greatly influencing modern Western social and cultural attitudes about how bodies *should* look, perform, and age. For example, a slender body symbolizes beauty, confidence, success, and willpower. In con-trast, a body that does not fit the thin ideal is stereotyped as unattract-ive, lazy, and uncontrollable. No matter one's body size, race, ability, gender, socioeconomic status, sexual orientation, or age, the constant stream of airbrushed images of celebrities and the headlines that ac-company them, unreasonable beauty ideals, a social fascination with "before and after" photos, fad diets, and quick-fix workouts leaves an impression.

Some people interpret these messages as motivational and others as shaming. Some respond neutrally, while others might feel annoyed or agitated from time to time. Some may experience varying degrees of self-consciousness or live with a generalized sense of "I am not good enough." Others may feel pressure to take extreme measures, like restricting their food intake, purging, or obsessively dieting. Some might compulsively body-check, weigh themselves, or exercise. Isolation, anxiety, depression, panic, and fear are all possible consequences of the dis-ease that accompa-nies negative body image.[1]

---

1. Sarah Grogan, *Body Image: Understanding Body Dissatisfaction in Men, Women, and Chil-dren* (New York: Routledge, 2016).

The cumulative effect of internalizing certain words and expressions in ways that undermine our self-worth and self-esteem can cause us to carry painful feelings about ourselves, endlessly seek validation from others, and fall into thinking and behavioral patterns that are physically and mentally detrimental. One of the major goals of this book is to help you become aware of how words positively or negatively influence your body image. After all, language shapes our reality, and therefore our words undoubtedly contribute to how we view our bodies.

The Power of Perception

What exactly is body image? According to Judy Lightstone, author of the article "Improving Body Image,"[2] body image involves our perception, imagination, emotions, and physical sensations of and about our bodies. Body image is sensitive to mood, environment, and physical experience. It is not based on fact; rather, it is learned in the family, among peers, and through social and cultural expectations.

Take a moment to fully take in the significance of these words: *body image is a perception and not a fact.* How does it feel to hear that your body image is not a fact? Respecting that statement as truth may very well be a life-altering moment, especially if you have experienced times of feeling bad about your body. Similarly, experiencing times of feeling good about your body is a powerful reminder of your ability to tap into self-affirming perceptions.

Perception is a way of regarding, understanding, or interpreting something; a mental impression. In this way, we can say our perceptions are a "body narrative" that we tell ourselves. Although our body narratives are strongly influenced by social messages, cultural expectations, and familial beliefs, they still belong to us, which means we have the capacity to challenge, shift, and reorient our perceptions about our bodies and all aspects of our lives, and, as you will learn over the course of this book, doing so begins with how we use and receive language.

---

2. Judy Lightstone, "Improving Body Image," Auckland PSI (Psycho Somatic Integration) Institute, http://www.psychotherapist.org/improving-body-image.html.

What awaits you in the pages that follow is a unique opportunity to study your relationship with your body with compassion and curiosity and glimpse how your language—the very words you think, speak, and absorb—informs your current body narrative, and then enhance or write new narratives that allow you to move through the world with an attitude that radiates self-confidence, self-empowerment, and peace.

The Pathway to Self-Empowerment

The goal of *Body Mindful Yoga* is to provide a foundation upon which you can create an affirming relationship with your body. We do not offer quick fixes, fad solutions, or empty promises. This is not a weight loss or diet book, and we also do not ask you to change your body in any way. Instead, *Body Mindful Yoga* is a book dedicated to helping you build the resolve to value your body through a transformational process founded on the principles of yoga. Chapter by chapter, you will learn how to nurture your ability to validate yourself and others. The way we feel about ourselves indirectly influences the way other people feel about themselves when they're around us. Self-respect and self-acceptance are contagious.

Our intention is to guide you to transform attitudes and beliefs that keep you stuck in disempowering body narratives about how you *should* look, perform, and age into self-affirming ones. Self-validation is not necessarily the response we are taught when it comes to body image, especially in a culture that thrives on external validation. The problem is that when we habitually rely on others to validate our worth, we never truly learn how to validate ourselves. As a result, we become enmeshed in guilt, shame, and comparison as we constantly strive to arrive at an ideal. The consequence is we lose sight of our unique qualities in exchange for external validation. We, the authors, understand this reality, as we both have lived it on various levels. However, we know there's a better, more fulfilling, and truthful way to be a member of society than to mirror values that cause us to underestimate our worth. This is the body mindful way. And it begins with our words.

Our inner dialogue—the words we say to ourselves and speak to others about our bodies—have tremendous power over our body image and self-esteem. Think for a moment: On days when you feel happy or upbeat, what's the quality of your thoughts about yourself? How about your vibe when you interact with others? In contrast, when you feel blah or low, what are you hearing in your mind? How is your mood expressed through your words and body language?

The exercises throughout this book will enlighten you to the relationship between your words and your body image. As you become more aware of how your inner language influences your own body image, you will also learn how to become more mindful of how your words can influence others to value their bodies in positive ways. As we will reiterate throughout this book, your words are powerful, so much so that not only do they have the potential to change the course of your relationship with your own body, but they can guide others to a more body-affirming life as well. The ripple effect that can begin by just one person being more mindful with their words is astoundingly profound!

Who Should Read This Book?

If you want to improve your confidence and reduce self-criticism, then this book is for you. After all, who doesn't have a little bit of room to show themselves more love, kindness, or respect? Take a moment and consider the highest qualities you value in a caring relationship with others. Which, if any, of those qualities do you honor for your body? If any are lacking, then this book is for you. The body mindful tools and practices will help you cultivate those highest qualities within yourself, for yourself.

Body Mindful Yoga is also for individuals who struggle with accepting their bodies. This book is a unique gateway to exploring body image, whether this is your first time looking at this topic in your own life or you have been working on it for years. The ideas and practices in this book can also easily complement therapeutic work around body image if you work with a therapist or other care provider.

This book is also a resource for therapists, social workers, and other healthcare professionals, as well as students and scholars who are interested in examining how language, social messages, and cultural expectations influence the human experience.

Body Mindful Yoga is for current and aspiring yoga practitioners as well. Although this book is focused specifically on the relationship between body image and language, the yogic lens through which we explore these topics offers a unique perspective. And, as yoga is a life practice, the lessons you may learn from this book are applicable to all realms of your existence.

Finally, we wish to emphasize that this book is designed to set readers on the path to a body-affirming life. When you reach the final page, your path will continue. The new insights you gain from this book will move you along your path in profound ways, no doubt. But, as in any relationship, it takes consistent daily effort to keep all parties involved content. The same goes for our relationship with our bodies. *Body Mindful Yoga* will best serve those of you who are committed to continuing on your personal path even after you complete reading the book. Affirming ourselves is a practice that takes daily effort, and the lessons and practices we provide here will give you a great foundation to continue on your body mindful journey.

What to Expect

Body Mindful Yoga presents a combination of yoga, social/cultural discourse, and self-reflection exercises—certainly a unique format for a book on body image! And as far as yoga books go, ours is also unique, teaching a variety of yoga-inspired wisdom and practices in the context of redefining your relationship with your body. We include many yoga poses, with instructions for how to perform them, as well as several types of mental, auditory, and visual yoga practices to accommodate your learning preferences. Yoga experience is not required to have a successful experience with this book; we will thoroughly guide you through every step.

In the opening chapters of the book, we discuss why language plays such an important role in determining how we feel about our bodies. We introduce you to the guiding principles of our body mindful philosophy and outline the Butera Method of Personal Transformation, a four-step method that adapts yoga philosophy for modern needs and is the foundation of the body mindful process presented in this book. The four steps—Listen, Learn, Love, and Live—will guide you to create and embody self-affirming body narratives.

The Listen and Learn steps are devoted to self-study, which in yoga refers to contemplation and reflection. In the Listen section, we guide you through exercises that ask you to reflect on your current feelings about your body and gain insight into where they came from. In the Learn section, we turn our attention to the role of language in forming body image. We examine four social facets (food, fitness, social media, and fashion) and some well-known slogans and expressions associated with each one. We also provide a chapter of additional slogan categories with suggested body mindful language that you can apply in other areas of your life. Ultimately, these chapters are designed to help you learn through personal reflection how certain words, expressions, and social messages influence you and then explore self-empowering ways to respond to them. We encourage you to work on those sections that are most applicable to your own life by focusing on the topics that are hot buttons for you. This way you will gain the most direct benefit from this process for your life and happiness.

The Love and Live sections bring to life the insights you gained in Listen and Learn through yoga practices to incorporate into your daily life. Think of the exercises in these sections as the glue that makes it all stick! We teach you how to apply body mindfulness to your inner life (the words you speak to yourself) through a variety of yoga practices and to your outer life (your interactions with others) by being a body mindful ambassador. You will learn how to listen and speak from a body mindful mindset, so that as you continue to empower and affirm yourself, you do the same for others as well.

Before We Get Started

We hope you will treat yourself to a new journal and keep it and a pen nearby. Use your journal to work through the exercises, record insights, and write freely about your feelings and past and present experiences.

The content in the Learn chapters is based on years of research and teaching yoga instructors about languaging. It is also inspired by the results of a survey we conducted in 2017–2018 in which two hundred men and women identified words, expressions, and slogans found in various facets of our society that influence their body image. Our goal is to give you the opportunity to learn if and how any of this language influences your body image and what shifts in perception could be helpful for developing an affirming body narrative. The Body Mindful Journaling exercises at the end of each chapter in this section will guide this self-reflection.

We wish to make clear our purposeful omission of sexual, racial, and vulgar comments and words related to physical ability. Although some of this language may influence your body image, our book is meant to be more general for you to apply in areas of your own life. Should that language come to light as you work through this book, we encourage you to get support and process your insights and emotional responses with trusted friends, family, clergy, or a therapist.

Our Personal Stories

Body Mindful Yoga was inspired by a variety of experiences in each of our lives. Although our stories are quite different, we share decades of personal and professional yoga experience and education and a passion for guiding others to self-learning that heals and empowers in the most momentous of ways. Here we share poignant moments from our personal stories and the work we've done in our own lives around language and body image. We, too, are works in progress in our ever-evolving relationships with our bodies, and we know firsthand that with commitment and practice, a body-affirming life is not only possible, but incredibly freeing.

Jennifer's Story

One of my fondest memories from college is of early-morning rowing practice.[3] In darkness and silence our team would run three miles from campus to the boathouse. Besides the occasional car that drove by, the

---

3. Some parts of my story were published in "When an Athlete Develops an Eating Disorder," *The Mighty*, September 14, 2016, https://themighty.com/2016/09/developing -an-eating-disorder-as-an-athlete.

only sound was the steady strike of feet on the pavement. Teams of eight and four would march their boats to the dock and set off on a moonlit river for a warm-up. We would power through drills as the sun came up, pushing and pulling to our maximum potential. It was a magical rhythm, this harmonious momentum we created with our bodies, oars, and the water.

Rowing is by far the most physically and mentally demanding sport I have ever participated in. I was the stroke for my boat and intensely driven to be a powerhouse rower. In grade school and high school, I played soccer, softball, and basketball. I excelled at all three sports and was named MVP most years. My goal was perfection: to score the most, win the most, and please my coaches and teammates. I practiced hard and played even harder. I prided myself on having a reputation for being aggressive. I craved the sweat, physical exertion, and glory of athleticism.

In my sophomore year of college, my drive for athletic success was challenged in a new and fierce way. During an afternoon rowing practice, as we rowed by the dock my coach shouted to our team, "I can tell how hard you work by how much your body changes." I remember how upon hearing his words I slammed down my legs and pulled the oars as hard as I possibly could. I had a new mission: to prove myself to my coach and team by changing my body. I interpreted my coach's words to mean that I had to shrink, for to become smaller would be the most visible way I could prove that my body had "changed." And, in the months to come, that's exactly what I did.

Before college I did not have a hypcrawareness of my body. I was average in size and comfortable in my skin. I was successful on the playing field with the body I had; I could box out with the best of them. Changing my body never occurred to me until that day on the water.

My coach's words—or, more accurately, the way I interpreted his words—unleashed a life-threatening eating disorder that severely altered my relationship with my body. I internalized my coach's words to mean that I must prove my worth through the size of my body, which became a complicated and deeply rooted core belief that I've devoted much of my life to unraveling. Now, more than twenty years later, I look back on that moment on the water and see so clearly the connection between language and body image: I let another's words get inside my head, infiltrate my spirit, interfere with my confidence, and ultimately distort my body image and self-esteem. And, as my internal dialogue grew darker, my mental health became more and more compromised.

My personal healing path led me to yoga, first as a practitioner, then as a teacher, and now as a certified Comprehensive Yoga Therapist with a specialty in eating disorders and body image. In June 2016 I had the good fortune of taking the position of Yoga Therapist at the Monte Nido Eating Disorder Center of Philadelphia in Villanova, Pennsylvania. Monte Nido, whose headquarters are in California, was the first eating disorder treatment center to include yoga in its clinical program. Monte Nido represented an extraordinary chance to hold space for others to heal their body image and self-esteem—a kind of healing I intimately knew was possible with yoga. As someone who has been through treatment for an eating disorder more than once, this opportunity also allowed me to give back to others in a unique and profound way.

In the weeks leading up to my first yoga therapy group at Monte Nido, I had the profound realization that I could not cue yoga poses there in the same way I had for years in my public yoga classes. I had a deep inner knowing that drawing attention to certain body parts could flare up an already acutely negative body image and disrupt any sense of calm and peace the clients were able to cultivate on the yoga mat. Therefore, if I wanted to create a safe space for these individuals, I needed to find new language to guide bodies in and out of yoga poses.

From that realization came the awareness that it was appropriate and necessary to extend this same sensitivity to students who attended my public yoga classes. After all, I didn't know what those individuals were contending with in their private lives in terms of body image, so why shouldn't I shift my language to support a body-affirming experience? So I stopped asking my students to reach higher, twist further, or sink lower. Instead, I honed my teaching to offer more options and variations so that students possessed the power of choice. I experimented with language that expressed a balance between challenging oneself and backing off in yoga poses. I found ways to use fewer (but not avoid) anatomical cues, especially for generally sensitive areas like the stomach and hips, and I experimented with a variety of approaches to guide an inner experience of sensation versus a physical one of overexertion. Essentially, I stopped asking others to prove themselves through their bodies.

I became so passionate about the need for sensitivity in my treatment and public yoga classes that I consulted with my friend and fellow yoga teacher and yoga therapist Erika Tenenbaum, as well as my primary yoga therapy teacher and coauthor, Bob Butera. Erika shared wonderful ideas about how to inspire curiosity in yoga students with language related to energy, color, shapes, and sensation. I shared my ideas with Bob and proposed creating a training in "body sensitivity" for yoga teachers, to which he responded, "Until we change the language within ourselves, we can't authentically help others heal."

Bob's wisdom swiftly set in motion the writing of this book. We had found a message that we needed to share with the world: *Change your language to heal your relationship with your body.* Our discussions inspired us to create the concept of *body mindful*, a unique approach that combines yoga and language for explaining, exploring, and healing negative body image.

My deepest hope is that *Body Mindful Yoga* will be a pathway to self-empowerment and a body-affirming life for all who strive to prove themselves through their bodies. May you find ease in your body and conviction in your words.

Bob's Story

"Yo, Ribs!" my first cousins would call to me. "Ribs" was slang for one of my Uncle Ray's affectionate nicknames for me, which was "Robs," short for "Robert Jr." With a Philly accent, it was easy for "Robs" to become "Ribs." It stuck because I was rail thin, or, as I liked to say, wiry strong. Even though most kids of my generation were skinny, I tended to be thinner than most. This nickname made me self-conscious of my protruding ribs.

Wanting to be tough, I didn't tell anyone that I hated the name Ribs. Instead, I did push-ups and sit-ups to beef up, and ate as much food as humanly possible, but I didn't gain any weight as a kid. I used this negative name to fuel my dominance as an athlete. Fortunately, I had above-average hand-eye coordination, so I was one of the best at all sports. I was one of the tougher kids probably because of my willpower combined with my advanced coordination. My athletic ability headed off the demeaning feeling of the nickname "Ribs," as I was also called "Sharpshooter," "Lefty," and just plain "Bobby" by the kids at school.

It's amazing how much those nicknames affected my childhood. Mind you, I was privileged in terms of my family having enough money for school and sports activities. Plus, I was intelligent and athletic. However, like all people, I had my trials.

From first to fourth grade, I carried the lunch tray of a boy who was permanently on crutches. I made sure that everyone at school treated him fairly and kindly. My friends all decided to accept him, and we didn't have any bullies in our homeroom, to my knowledge.

The protector in me, however, cannot protect any of us from the word structures in our minds. Ideas like fear, guilt, and shame are embedded in our very thought patterns. Language holds these patterns in rigid form. This book is a way to help you see your own patterns in a friendly and down-to-earth way. With self-awareness, you may be able to better understand yourself and make huge strides forward.

I was also very advanced in mathematics as a kid, but my English skills were average. Ideas formed so quickly in my mind that I couldn't find the words to express them fast enough. And when I did speak quickly, most people couldn't follow my ideas. Fortunately, my mother highly valued listening skills. Her patience saved me. She taught me the power of permitting someone to develop and express their thoughts. I have always valued the benefits of being heard. I think few of us are truly listened to, and hence, we aren't very good at listening to ourselves. And then we aren't very good at undoing or changing the way we speak to ourselves. With this book, I hope to help you determine your baseline—your current relationship with your body—by listening within. This step alone could be the key for you to recognize what changes could maximize your potential.

During my time at a very liberal (in terms of feminism) liberal arts college in Japan, one of my best teachers was actually a classmate, a self-declared feminist who went out of her way to inform others that being a feminist did not mean she was angry at men. She sought to refute the assumption that feminism was associated with anger. My peer taught me that language represents internal states of mind, and that most of us are unaware of how our words reflect values we might not even understand, which became even clearer when I learned to speak Chinese and Japanese. The nuances of those languages revealed to me many of my own patterns and how my language had shaped my life experiences. Speaking foreign languages fluently taught me that language itself had the power to alter my personality and feelings toward life. With Japanese, I felt very proper, very regimented, very exact. Chinese was more fluid to me, easygoing and somewhat mystical because of the loose grammatical rules.

As I continued my education at other liberal graduate schools, I met many more feminists who helped me recognize archaic thought patterns that exist in my consciousness to this day. I have learned to accept that culture affects me and to some degree controls my ability to reason. I continue to learn and let others be my teachers.

People call me "YogaBob" at our institute, and others say "Dr. Bob." Some who know me as a surfer call me "Shreddy." Ribs, Robs, Bobby, Uncle, and all my other names affect me far less these days. I have developed some ability to filter messages from the outer world versus letting nicknames define me. I can define myself from within.

Discussions with Jennifer, my coauthor, have rekindled my interest in the relationship between language and enlightenment. How can I be enlightened if the English language holds my thoughts in grammatical structures and in word meanings? Even though I spoke fluently in Canadian French, Chinese, and Japanese during the times I lived in those countries, English still grips my waking thoughts.

Mystics say that union with the divine begins where words end. I have experienced deep states of mystical prayer. These peak experiences and other strong feelings of higher connection are temporary, and I fall back into a waking consciousness whereby my English words still reflect a division from reality.

My personal goal with *Body Mindful Yoga* is to hold words lightly, to not take my ideas too seriously, so that I speak more softly and more patiently. This way, I can shape English around my deeper values and control language's effect on me. Once I can do this, I will be a good ambassador for my friends and loved ones. If our work inspires you to feel freer to affirm yourself and makes you a better person, then please share your gifts with others to bring more love into the world.

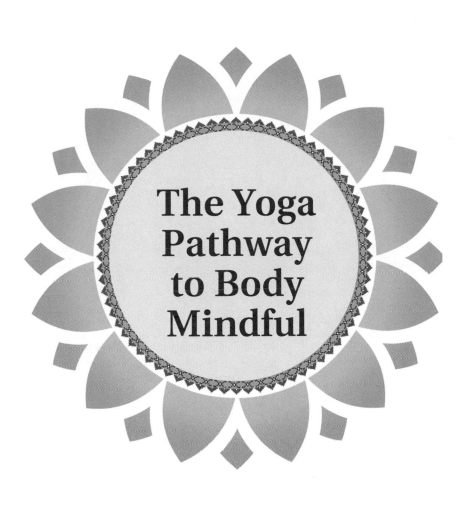

The Yoga
Pathway
to Body
Mindful

The opening chapters of this book explain why language plays such an important role in determining how we feel about our bodies. We introduce you to the guiding principles of our body mindful philosophy, the essence of which is to enlighten you to how language influences your body image and to teach you to speak mindfully about your body. We discuss *body narratives*, the stories we tell ourselves about our bodies, and how guilt, shame, and comparison entrap us in disempowering body narratives. We also teach how reliance on external validation reinforces disempowering body narratives. We outline the Butera Method of Personal Transformation, the four-step method that adapts yoga philosophy for modern needs and is the foundation of the body mindful process presented in this book. The four steps—Listen, Learn, Love, and Live—will guide you to develop affirming and self-empowering body narratives and teach you how to incorporate body mindful yoga practices and rituals into your daily life.

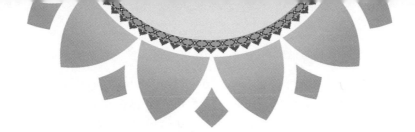

Chapter 1

Understanding Language and the Narratives We Tell

This chapter introduces you to two key concepts: *body mindful* and *body narratives*. We begin by describing how yoga philosophy guides us to look inward rather than outward for validation. We define body mindful and outline the guiding principles of this concept. We share statistics about body dissatisfaction among adults and adolescents, and discuss body narratives—where they come from, how they work, and how to rewrite the parts that are disempowering and celebrate the parts that are affirming.

Words Are Our Greatest Source of Personal Power

Yoga philosophy teaches that we have everything we need inside of us to tend to all of life's moments, from the happiest to the most challenging ones. When we slow down, get quiet, and pay attention to our personal wisdom, we can gain tremendous clarity about what we need to improve a situation, make a decision, or solve a problem. In other words, all the answers we seek exist inside of us already; we need only trust in our ability to access them.

This philosophy counters our overly stimulating consumer-driven culture. As a society, we are conditioned to look outside of ourselves for answers, seeking external validation for our decisions, feelings, and dreams. We are taught to go faster, push harder, buy more, follow others' advice, keep up with trends, chase an ideal. We also turn outward for others' approval of our bodies. We do this directly with questions like *Do I look all right?* or *How do I look?* and indirectly when we compare ourselves to others, including images on social media and in magazines. Comparison is always a moment of looking outside of ourselves for a sign that we are "okay." In the words of Theodore Roosevelt, "Comparison is the thief of joy." When we define ourselves according to external standards rather than internal ones, we never truly stand in our personal power.

One of the most profound ways we lose hold of our personal power is through our language, especially when we negate instead of affirm, belittle instead of empower, chastise instead of validate ourselves. Our language is everything: it shapes our reality, reinforces our body image, and reflects how we feel about ourselves. How we absorb or internalize others' words and how we speak to ourselves directly impacts our body image and self-esteem.

Our language is not separate from our bodies; the two are intimately connected. Our bodies translate language through mood, health, perception, and disposition. For example, when we tell ourselves that we don't measure up, that attitude comes through in subtle ways in our bodies. We might hunch our shoulders or not look others in the eye. This attitude will likely influence how we dress and maybe even how we look at food and nourish our bodies. In contrast, when we feed our minds words of confidence, we are likely to stand a little taller, feel more entitled to share our ideas, and be less distracted by what others are doing. Our dress probably mirrors our confidence, and we're less likely to compare ourselves to others. The good news is that we can regain our personal power by using language purposefully and mindfully. This is a foundational belief of our body mindful philosophy.

Introducing Body Mindful: What Does It Mean?

Body mindful means to speak mindfully about your body. Body mindfulness is to purposely choose words that nurture self-validation and affirm your body in your self-talk and conversations with others. To be body mindful means to intentionally refrain from disparaging body talk and to challenge guilt, shame, and comparison self-talk. When we are body mindful, we trust that we do not need to measure ourselves against others or change our bodies in the name of social or beauty ideals. Ultimately, body mindful is a pathway to the gifts and answers that already exist inside of us, those virtues like confidence, resilience, courage, hope, appreciation, and grace that empower us from the inside out and allow us to embrace an attitude of possibility. We can strive to change our exteriors over and over again, but unless our insides are aligned with our higher selves (all of those beautiful virtues), we will never know how to affirm our bodies.

Guiding Principles of Body Mindful

Body mindful consists of three guiding principles:

1. Our desire for external validation plays out in our relationship with our body, which includes how we hold it, dress it, feed it, describe it, perceive it, and respect it, and how we view others' bodies.
2. Our language either nurtures self-validation in ourselves and others or feeds the desire for external validation.
3. Our relationship with our body is affirming when we rely on self-validation instead of external validation.

These guiding principles are the backbone of the body mindful philosophy. The transformational work in the chapters that follow will open your eyes to your own body-language relationship and give you some practice decoding disempowering words and messages. You will learn how to be purposeful with your words and responsible for your body image. Body mindful puts this power in your hands.

Body Narratives

Have you ever felt pressured to prove your worth through your body, be it through size or shape, speed or strength, fashion sense, or physical features such as height or hair color and length? In the moments when we feel we "passed" the test, that our bodies performed adequately, we may feel proud, happy, gratified, or relieved. On the opposite end of the spectrum, when we feel "less than," feelings of inadequacy may snowball into varying degrees of guilt, shame, and comparison.[4,5] Guilt is a focus on a behavior and evokes the feeling that "I did something bad." Shame is a focus on the self and is expressed as "I am bad." We use comparison to determine our personal and social worth based on our perception of others, the past, or the future. Comparison thinking can fuel "I am not good enough" beliefs, which contribute to low self-esteem and poor body image. These heavy feelings often show up when we feel compelled to compete with the "ideal" bodies on display throughout our social universe.

If you can relate, we offer you the comfort of knowing you are far from alone. According to Dr. Margo Maine, concern with body appearance significantly affects girls' and women's academic and professional performance and intellectual functioning. According to research presented by Dr. Maine in 2017 at the National Eating Disorder Information Centre's Body Image and Self-Esteem Conference, 15% of girls reportedly skip school, 13% will not speak out to give an opinion, 5% will not go to a job interview, and 3% will call out of work when they feel bad about their bodies. Similarly, 17% of women reportedly will not show up for a job interview, and 8% will not go to work.[6]

In 2016 the journal *Body Image* reported a high prevalence of body dissatisfaction among adults in the United States.[7] The study, which in-

---

4. *Shame Verses [sic] Guilt—Brene' Brown,* YouTube, Jan Fleury channel, Sept. 21, 2015, https://www.youtube.com/watch?v=DqGFrId-IQg.

5. Michael J. Formica, "Negative Self-Perception and Shame," *Psychology Today,* July 24, 2008, https://www.psychologytoday.com/us/blog/enlightened-living/200807/negative-self-perception-and-shame.

6. Margo Maine, "Invisible Women: Eating Disorders and the Pressure to Be Perfect at Midlife and Beyond: A Relational Culture Approach," National Eating Disorder Information Centre (NEDIC), http://nedic.ca/node/976.

7. David A. Frederick, Gaganjyot Sandhu, Patrick J. Morse, and Viren Swami, "Correlates of Appearance and Weight Satisfaction in a U.S. National Sample: Personality, Attachment Style, Television Viewing, Self-Esteem, and Life Satisfaction," *Body Image* 17 (June 2016): 191–203, https://doi.org/10.1016/j.bodyim.2016.04.001.

cluded 12,176 US men and women who completed an online survey, found that only about a quarter of the participants were satisfied with their appearance.

The 2017 Dove Global Girls Beauty and Confidence Report, which interviewed 5,165 girls aged 10 to 17 across 14 countries, reported that higher levels of body esteem have a lasting impact on a girls' confidence, resilience, and life satisfaction.[8] Conversely, poor body image was associated with not participating in social activities due to feeling self-conscious about their appearance. The report found that girls generally would prefer that the media include more diverse body sizes and are dissatisfied with the emphasis on beauty as a means of happiness.

These statistics illuminate the potentially all-consuming nature of a negative body image. They also tell a story in which confidence, assertiveness, and other self-empowering qualities are overshadowed by despairing beliefs of not measuring up, taking up too much space, always falling short, never being thin enough, and so on. Such beliefs form our body narratives, the stories we tell ourselves about our bodies and the things we say to ourselves about how our bodies look, feel, compare, and fit in. Your narrative might play on repeat or pop in and out of your mind less frequently. You may have multiple narratives about your body that kick in depending on where you are or what you are doing. For example, how you feel in your body while you're playing sports, walking in the park, or sitting in your favorite comfy chair may be entirely different from when you're at a family gathering or a doctor's appointment. That's because each of these scenarios comes with its own set of dynamics, expectations, and histories that consciously and subconsciously influence how you hold, dress, feed, describe, perceive, and treat your body. All this information merges together to create your body narrative(s).

Although our body narratives are strongly influenced by social messages and cultural expectations, they still belong to us, which means we

---

8. "Girls on Beauty: New Dove Research Finds Low Beauty Confidence Driving 8 in 10 Girls to Opt Out of Future Opportunities," PRNewswire, October 5, 2017, https://www.prnewswire.com/news-releases/girls-on-beauty-new-dove-research-finds-low-beauty-confidence-driving-8-in-10-girls-to-opt-out-of-future-opportunities-649549253.html.

have the capacity to challenge and reorient unhelpful perceptions. As in any good story, ups and downs are to be expected. Yet we, the authors of our personal body narratives, have complete and total control over the writing of our stories. We have the potential to transform the body narratives that hold us back. *You* have the power to redefine your relationship with your body, and the exercises in the upcoming chapters will put you on the path to beginning that transformational work.

Chapter Summary

1. Yoga teaches that we suffer less when we define ourselves from within and let go of relying on external validation.

2. Language shapes our reality and how we view ourselves.

3. These are the three guiding principles of our body mindful philosophy:

    • Our desire for external validation plays out in our relationship with our body, which includes how we hold it, dress it, feed it, describe it, perceive it, and respect it, and how we view others' bodies.

    • Our language either nurtures self-validation in ourselves and others or feeds the desire for external validation.

    • Our relationship with our body is affirming when we rely on self-validation instead of external validation.

4. Language includes nonverbals, namely body posture and facial expressions.

5. Our bodies translate language through mood, health, perception, and disposition.

6. Identifying negative self-talk rooted in guilt, shame, and comparison empowers you to replace undermining language with positive, internally based statements.

7. Guilt means "I did something bad."

8. Shame means "I am bad."

9. Comparison is when we determine our personal and social worth based on our perception of others, the past, or the future.

10. You have the power to overcome self-limiting views with self-empowering words.

11. Body narratives are the stories we tell ourselves about our bodies.

12. As the author of your personal body narratives, you have complete and total control over your story and the power to transform the beliefs that hold you back.

This chapter taught you about the fundamental ideas and philosophies upon which this book is built, the main ideas being that your words hold great influence and you can use your language as a source of personal empowerment. By studying your habits, specifically when you use disempowering language rooted in guilt, shame, and comparison, you can begin to learn why you do so and then set your mind to creating new, more affirming ways of speaking about yourself, strengthening your body image and sense of self along the way.

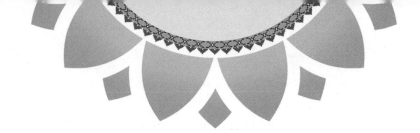

Chapter 2

Four Steps on the Path:
Listen, Learn, Love, Live

So often we desire change but either fear the idea of change itself or believe it to be unattainable. The more we wish for something to be different, the more we suffer. We become anxious, ruminate, grow resentful, and maybe even experience moments of hopelessness. Social messages endeavor to convince us that we will *finally* be fulfilled once we physically change our bodies and that the answer to personal happiness exists outside of us, like in a diet or the number on the scale. But lasting change is only possible when we unravel the beliefs that led us to believe we weren't good enough in the first place and then look inside for the answer we seek.

The Butera Method of Personal Transformation and Finding Your Starting Point

The Butera Method of Personal Transformation is a pathway to meaningful change because you get to be an active participant in each step. Your main task is to learn about yourself and then convert that new wisdom into body mindfulness in your life. There is no cost involved, and there are no diets to try or fitness fads to burn out on. Instead, the key to creating change in your relationship with your body is first to find your starting point—the foundation upon which all four steps of the Butera Method will build.

Bob began creating this method thirty years ago. Here he shares that story and outlines the four steps that will support you in making lasting body mindful changes in your own life.

Quest for Enlightenment

"He likes everything different," my grandmother said after I (Bob) returned home from Asia with a big beard and conversationally fluent in Japanese and Chinese. In the latter half of the 1980s, I traveled abroad to French-speaking Quebec, Canada, Europe, Japan, Taiwan, and India, with a flurry of short trips to places like Hong Kong, Thailand, South Korea, Scotland, Switzerland, and France. My quest was to become enlightened in every aspect of life. I also longed to figure out how to use my life to make the world a more peaceful place. I was curious, hungry to learn and experience better ways of living. Even as a child, I was always examining the status quo, questioning and testing everything. My grandmother didn't realize that although I had learned all sorts of meaningful things from her and so many other wise individuals in my life, I still wanted more knowledge. Being the consummate student of every area of life prepared me to become the teacher I am today.

During my studies at the Yoga Institute in Mumbai, India, yoga captivated me. This system of thought incorporated all aspects of life that I wished to study, both enlightenment within myself and positive human relationships with others. In the 1930s, the institute's founder, Sri Yogendra (1897–1989), defined yoga education as a complete mastery of consciousness. I remember Shri Yogendra describing yoga education in a lecture toward the end of his life as "an education of the total human being." Yoga education, which is very different from a typical yoga class of poses, teaches us how to address our emotional, spiritual, physical, and intellectual health simultaneously. I was exhilarated by the idea that all dimensions of our human experience could be studied through this single lens. Rather than taking the traditional academic approach of separating disciplines of study, like psychology, religion, and physiology, yoga education considers, values, and incorporates each aspect of life. For example, nutritional education considers the food you eat as well as how you eat it, with whom you eat it, and why you eat it. Exercise education includes the obvious physical component but also teaches how and why a person's internal mindset is equally important.

The four steps of yoga education—duty, realized knowledge, non-attachment, and mastery—are derived from a branch of Indian philosophy called *Samkhya*. As archaic as that word may sound, so too are the names of the four steps that make up yoga education. Duty, or *dharma*, is related to our priorities and roles in life, including responsibilities to self, family and friends, work, society, and all of humanity. Knowledge, or *jnana*, refers to physical, emotional, and spiritual self-awareness. Non-attachment, or *vairagya*, is to view our lives as an objective witness, to live with our struggles but not be defined by them. Mastery, or *Ishvara aishvarya*, refers to a humble feeling of achievement, satisfaction, and knowledge that can arise from applying duty, knowledge, and non-attachment to one's life.

These yogic terms, while filled with wisdom, don't necessarily sound so catchy in today's world, but they banged around in my head for thirty years. Yes, thirty years! I knew these concepts inside and out. I taught and wrote about them extensively; they were vital components of the transformational learning method I taught in trainings and seminars.

I couldn't put my finger on it, but something about these concepts was missing for my modern-day Western students. Little did I know back then, as a student in India, that these vital concepts from yoga philosophy would be the building blocks of the four-step program for transformational learning I'd develop for the Western student called the Butera Method of Personal Transformation.

From Frustration to Inspiration

The Butera Method came together in the wake of what seems to happen to me roughly once every three years: I deliver a lecture that falls flat and doesn't fulfill the audience's needs. I can recall five talks that earned standing ovations at one venue but garnered less-than-flattering feedback at another setting. The following story is the best example of this, because from its ashes was born the Butera Method of Personal Transformation.

A talk I had given twenty times before to smaller groups was preceded by a few red flags: The staff didn't know which room I was to be in; the starting time was off by thirty minutes; five minutes before the start time I was asked if the talk was open to the public or just the training group; and, to top it off, I was told the length of the seminar had been reduced from two hours to ninety minutes. All of this happened while I was being directed to the wrong room.

Once everyone was settled, I asked the group of seventy yoga teachers and practitioners to reflect on what archetypes meant to them. An *archetype* is defined as an original model or type after which other similar things are patterned. An archetype may be derived from but not limited to elements found in nature, mythological stories, spiritual symbols, aspects of character, geometric patterns, and certain words. The group's eyes glazed over in disinterest as I explained the definition of an archetype. As I looked out at the group of blank faces, I secretly imagined that at any minute I'd get "the hook" and be dragged off the stage like a bad comedian.

Clearly this audience was expecting something that I was not delivering, yet I pushed on. Just as the seminar description had promised, I enthusiastically explained how yoga poses may be performed from an archetypal perspective. Blank stares continued for the first ten minutes of the ninety-minute program. It was not going well, to say the least.

I tried a visualization exercise that I had used many times before. People fidgeted. One staffer left. Another thought I was a rookie. I was as surprised as anyone, but the audience didn't know that I had given this talk twenty times previously with extraordinary results.

Next, I suggested that we just try a yoga pose and see how it went. I asked the group to stand up and raise their arms overhead. Suddenly notebooks opened and eyes twinkled as I explained how a pose works from an archetypal perspective. I hate to admit it, but my talking was turning people off. A few confused smiles were trying to tell me, "Silly man, all we want to learn are some unique how-tos and teaching cues for yoga poses." And so I threw out my plan and showed the group several poses that I knew would intrigue them. As I guided them in and out of yoga poses with physical cues that were new to them, things smoothed over. Blank stares turned enthusiastic, but the group never grasped the concept of archetypes.

A year later, after giving fifty engaging book tour seminars, I hit this sort of blank-stare wall again. This time, though, I was less surprised by the students' lost reaction to my lecture. This group of eighteen wanted me to tell them how to feel and what to do. Obviously, my teaching method of inquiry and student empowerment was confusing matters. I couldn't seem to get across the point of archetypes the way I had in other venues.

Like before, I had the group start moving in yoga poses. This time I asked the students questions to guide their movements and invited them to answer out loud. At first the questions confused them, but now I was in my comfort zone of inquiry, so I coached the group on how to listen with patience. "Where is your attention right now?" I asked. To their surprise, answers started flowing. Most of the students in the room had similar answers. They were all focused on an area of their body that their yoga instructors frequently talked about when they did this particular pose in their daily classes.

Next I asked, "What are your eyes doing?" This question sparked a variety of answers. Some students said they looked up, and others said straight ahead. One woman said her eyes were closed. I continued with this inquiry exercise: "Where is your breath? What do you feel physically? How about emotionally?" Self-reflection in yoga poses was a completely new experience for this group.

After fifteen minutes, the group was hungry for more questions. The students were learning things about themselves that they had never considered. I rolled with it for another fifteen minutes, having people share answers with the group to show the variety of perspectives that each person held but didn't seem to know they did. We covered a series of poses, and I drilled them with questions. Patterns emerged for each person. For example, the guy who mentioned his tight low back noticed that he obsessed about his back in every pose. The woman intent on feeling her emotions kept explaining how different poses connected to her heart. The very muscular triathlete noticed that she was focused on coordinating her breath with movement.

Their insights led to more questions, which led to more insights. One woman shared, "That blows my mind! Now I know why I can't do this pose a certain way: it doesn't suit me." Another said, "I never realized that I was doing everything from my heart chakra." Another person finally came to realize that she felt dizzy when doing yoga because she was always looking around the room, worried about whether she was doing it correctly. The students shared that they had learned more about themselves and their personal approach to yoga poses in that thirty-minute spontaneous exercise than they had in years of yoga classes.

The group learned about archetypes in the final forty-five minutes of the seminar. From that moment on, I have led my seminars in this way: first I lead the group in inquiry exercises for discovering personal insights and then I introduce the new topic.

Finally, the Missing Piece!

These two workshop experiences revealed to me the essential step in the transformational learning method I'd been unofficially teaching based on the four steps of yoga education. Finally, after thirty years, it all came together in this one essential principle: *Know where you are now to make the next step count.*

I realized how every teacher I had ever had, from childhood through graduate school and beyond, had introduced new information in class without really exploring or understanding my own personal starting point in relation to the material. The one exception was when I received Yoga Therapy and the teacher was focused on me. Like the teachers before me, I taught the same way: I presented a topic for students to learn without carving out time for them to examine their own self-understanding in relation to that topic. These two workshops (and any class I've ever taught that was not so well received) were clear indicators of how important it is for students to see themselves in relation to the content before taking in new information.

From this realization was born the four-step program for transformational learning called the Butera Method of Personal Transformation. This method is designed to help you make meaningful changes in your life by actively transforming perspectives and behaviors in ways that are authentic and appropriate to your learning style.

Next, we will outline the four steps and describe how each one will serve you on your body mindful journey.

The Four Steps

The Butera Method of Personal Transformation adapts yoga philosophy for modern students' needs. The four steps are the foundation of the body mindful process we will begin in the next chapter. Here are the four steps:

1. Listen: Know thyself.

Study your strengths and weaknesses to determine where you are in your life and identify what you need your next step to be. Naming a starting point allows you to chart a course for future success.

2. Learn: Honor what you know and invite new wisdom.

Now that you are clearly aware of your starting point, dive into learning what you need to empower yourself to serve others and be at peace within.

3. Love: Practice new wisdom in your inner life.

To embody knowledge is to practice it in your personal life and in your mind. Notice how words fill your mind in different situations. Practice using words carefully in your yoga, meditation, creative, and other personal practices. You will be able to measure your progress as new situations arise.

4. Live: Share new wisdom with others through example.
Model affirming language for others so you empower others as well as yourself.

These four steps will open your eyes to how words affect your body image. The first two steps, Listen and Learn, are reflection-based. In yoga, we call this self-study. In these two steps you will uncover nuances about your relationship with your body and how your language shapes your body image. The last two steps, Love and Live, are practice-based. This means you will learn how to incorporate exercises and rituals into your daily life that support a self-affirming relationship with your body.

Let's get started!

Chapter Summary

1. Yoga education considers all dimensions of a person during the learning process, including their emotional, spiritual, physical, and intellectual health.

2. The Butera Method of Personal Transformation is based on the yoga philosophy concepts of duty, knowledge, non-attachment, and mastery.

3. This method is designed to help you make meaningful changes in your life by actively transforming perspectives and behaviors in ways that are authentic and appropriate to your learning style.

4. The four steps are a road map for developing an affirming relationship with your body, with the first step focused on identifying a solid starting point from which to grow.

5. Here are the four steps:
   - Listen: Know thyself. Know your strengths and weaknesses.
   - Learn: Honor what you know and invite new wisdom.
   - Love: Practice new wisdom in your inner life.
   - Live: Share new wisdom with others through example.

6. The first two steps (Listen and Learn) are focused on personal reflection, and the last two steps (Love and Live) are practice-oriented,

giving you hands-on tools and exercises to incorporate into your daily life.

Now that you understand the Butera Method of Personal Transformation, we'll move on to the first step: Listen. In the next chapter you will examine how you think about your body and yourself in different situations in your life and chart a course for strengthening your relationship with your body.

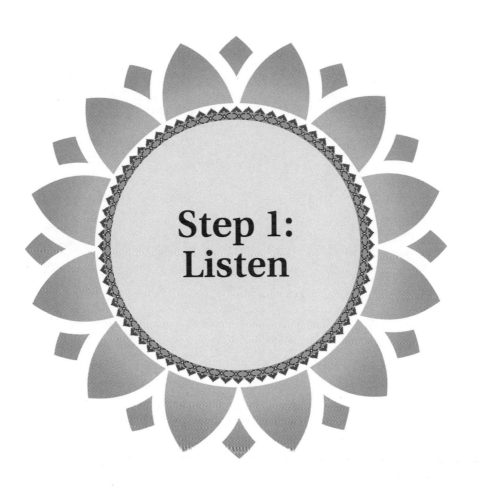

Step 1:
Listen

Welcome to Listen, the first step of the Butera Method of Personal Transformation. In this chapter you will establish your body mindful baseline (meaning where you are right now in your relationship with your body) and identify body mindful goals for how you want that relationship to change or shift. You will also examine the factors that influence your body image. The other exercises in this chapter will focus on getting to know your body narrative(s) and learning how to use the yogic practice of intention setting to support your body mindful journey.

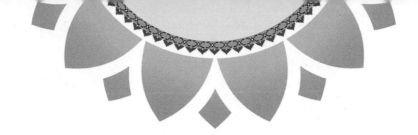

Chapter 3
Know Thyself

Your experiences are rich with wisdom about how you currently relate to your body. The exercises and ideas in this chapter will give you an opportunity to extract the lessons from your experiences and then set body mindful goals and an intention to guide your steps throughout this book.

Life's Tests Are Lessons in the Making

The phrase "wax on, wax off" was made famous by Kesuke Miyagi, fondly known as Mr. Miyagi in the 1984 American martial arts film *The Karate Kid*. The karate master begins his student Daniel's karate lessons with arduous chores like waxing cars, sanding a wooden floor, refinishing a fence, and painting Mr. Miyagi's house. Each task is accomplished with a specific hand motion. In the memorable "wax on, wax off" scene, Mr. Miyagi teaches Daniel to wax his collection of antique cars with distinct circular motions for each hand. Daniel is perplexed, confused, and angry, because he visits Mr. Miyagi to learn karate, not wax his cars or work odd jobs. Days later Daniel learns that the circular movements are defensive moves for blocking strikes.

Ancient masters and great teachers like Mr. Miyagi devise learning experiences for the student to figure out the meaning of a lesson completely on their own. By teaching through challenging tasks, teachers strive to ignite the quest for learning in the student. Giving freedom to the student to invent their learning process is both dangerous and powerful—dangerous because if you overstep the student's capabilities, the student may give up or rebel out of frustration, and powerful because when a person figures something out on their own, they "own" it. When we own our lessons, we are empowered, because we have a gut feeling about what is right. We do not need another person's recommendation or blessing.

Without any knowledge of the significance of why he was waxing his master's car, Daniel felt all sorts of emotions. The teacher's goal in this situation was to expose Daniel's underlying personality strengths and weaknesses that would be revealed when he was under duress. It was meant to reveal Daniel's natural reactions to confusion and obstacles. Before he could compete as a proficient martial artist and eventually become a champion, Daniel first had to become aware of his natural instincts, understand his strengths and weaknesses, and get clear about his goals and motivations. He had to first *listen* to the thoughts and beliefs that were obstacles to his concentration and commitment before he could move forward and feel truly empowered as a young man and martial artist.

Of course, real life is very different from what we see in movies. In *The Karate Kid*, the camera jumps ahead, so we don't have to watch every minute of Daniel's trying days of waxing, sanding, and painting. In our personal lives, this sort of test is not as easy to watch, as we star in the lead role, which never ends. There are no commercial breaks. But this is a gift, because our every experience is a lesson in the making, and the best way to succeed at life's tests is to know where you are now in order to make the next step count. We can create meaningful change in our lives if we identify a starting point. This also applies to valuing our bodies. The first step in knowing where you are in your relationship to your body is to listen—to turn inward and get a sense of what we call your body mindful baseline.

What's Your Body Mindful Baseline?

Let's establish a baseline, or starting point. Your baseline is your current relationship with your body. This starting point is influenced by multiple factors, and, if you are willing to listen to your inner wisdom, the exercises in this chapter will enlighten you to the truth of where you are now and what you need in order to take the next step in improving your body image. Your replies may lead to some of the most significant insights you gain from this entire book. Be honest. Be blunt. Don't hesitate. Listen to your gut and write down what it tells you. If writing in a journal is not your preference, simply reflect on the answers in your mind or return to this exercise when you feel ready.

EXERCISE: Your Body Narrative

Step 1: This exercise is the first of many in this book that will ask you to examine how your words affect your self-esteem, your love, your compassion, your sense of beauty, and your identity. Grab a journal and take a listen within by answering a few questions. There's no right format for your answers. There's nothing to hide. Let the words flow. This is just for you.

- How do people in your life talk about their bodies?
- How do you describe your body?
- What is your definition of a healthy body?
- Who or what influences your definition of a healthy body?
- What is your definition of a beautiful body?
- Who or what influences your definition of a beautiful body?
- What do you like about your body?
- What do you not like about your body?
- What is your relationship to your body? How do you treat it? For example, are you caring, kind, neutral, self-deprecating, dismissive, disdainful, etc.?
- In your heart of hearts, how do you wish to feel about your body?

Step 2: Continue to listen within and write your *body narrative*, the story you carry with you about your body based on your answers to the previous questions. A body narrative is made up of the memories, words, and emotions you hear in your mind and/or say out loud to others about your body. It can be as short or as long as you like. Give yourself the time and space to get this out—it's important to *listen* to yourself. Do your best not to edit or censor yourself. Let the words flow.

Here are two fictitious examples to give you an idea of what we mean:

Joe's Body Narrative: I am a fifty-three-year-old man. I was overweight until my mom put me on a diet when I was thirteen, and I have stayed thin ever since. I have been told how good I look, especially by my childhood friends who remember when I was overweight. I have felt so much better about myself since that time. But if I were taller, things would be even better. I am not very tall, and there isn't much I can do about it. Still, I would have made the varsity football and baseball teams if I had been bigger. Now that I think about it, although I have never talked about it, I have a big nose. No one says anything, but I know it's true. Because of my flaws, I am very kind and sensitive to others and never want anyone to feel bad about their body. I guess I'm a nice guy because I know the feeling of being less than others.

Michelle's Body Narrative: I am twenty-six and don't really have anything positive to say about my body. I am trying to find a new job. I was fortunate to be able to go to a good college, and I do have a job now, but it's not very fulfilling. I feel self-conscious when I go on interviews because I feel really fat. I know I am average-size, but I feel like average isn't good enough. I am curvy and probably bigger than average. I think if I could lose some weight, I would feel more confident at interviews. I'd also feel more deserving of a relationship. My parents were always critical of my body, so sometimes I feel ashamed of how I look when I go out. I find it's much more comfortable to stay home than to be social. I'm just always haunted by this feeling of not being good enough.

Step 3: Read through your body narrative. Underline or circle words and phrases that strike you. Take some time for self-study and write in your journal about your reactions to your body narrative. Consider these questions: How do you feel reading your words? What emotions come up? Where do you feel these emotions in your body?

Step 4: Write out or list the ripple effects of your body narrative. In other words, how does the way you feel about your body affect all facets of your life, such as your relationships, career, social interactions, spiritual life, mental health, physical health, and self-confidence? Be honest and also gentle with yourself. We understand how listening to our truth can be uncomfortable. We also know that such self-study can lead to breakthroughs that put us on a life-changing path that's been waiting for us all along.

EXERCISE: What Influences Your Body Image?

Now that you've studied your body narrative, let's look at the factors that contributed to forming it. Several major influences shape our perceptions and beliefs about our bodies and self-worth from the time we are small children. Skim this list and notice which categories jump out as important for your personal experience. Make notes in your journal or in the margins of this book about how some of these factors have influenced your thoughts and beliefs about your body. You might also jot down childhood nicknames or other relevant words from your past.

Family
Mother/female guardian
Father/male guardian
Grandparents
Influential family members and elders
Siblings
Birth order

Peer Pressure
Friends
Social engagement (clubs, sports, hobbies)
Social media

Community
Cultural expectations (school)
Religious expectations (personal/family spiritual experience)

Physical Response to Thinking About Your Body Image
Body posture
Tense areas of your body
Breathing pattern
Emotional state
Facial expression

Create a Body Mindful Goal

Now that you've spent some time reflecting on the words you use to describe your body and the influential factors that have shaped how you think about your body, let's go inward again.

EXERCISE: Set Your Body Mindful Goals

Listen to the thoughts that come up in response to this question: *What are your goals for your body?* Follow the three steps outlined here to complete this exercise.

Step 1: List your body goals. These can be past or current goals about health, weight, shape, and size. They can be goals for health, athleticism, or exercise. Any goal that is related to your body or an attribute of it can go on this list. You can also include fantasies about how your life would change if only you had a different body, as these thoughts tend to subconsciously influence our body goals.

Step 2: Review your list of body goals. Mark which ones empower versus disempower you.

For example, an empowering body mindful goal might be this: *My goal is to feel energetic.* This statement is empowering because it expresses a positive feeling that supports your health.

A disempowering goal might be this: *My goal is to lose ten pounds so I can look like my neighbor.* This goal is disempowering because it is based on comparison to the neighbor. The problem with this statement is the emphasis on "fixing" your body to look like someone else's.

Step 3: Identify one empowering body mindful goal that you wish to manifest in your life. This can be one that you listed in step 1 or a brand-new one. What's most important is that this goal uses positive, uplifting language.

For example, an empowering body mindful goal might be this: *My goal is to stand tall and look people in the eye when I speak.*

Here is an example of a body mind*less* goal: *My goal is to buy expensive clothing so people will think I am put together and accomplished.*

Here are a few additional examples of body mindful goals:

• *My goal is to feel energetic.*
• *My goal is to enjoy health.*
• *My goal is to build stamina.*
• *My goal is to improve my cardiovascular health.*
• *My goal is to enjoy exercise in nature.*
• *My goal is to have more energy to play with my children/grandchildren.*
• *My goal is to feel more alive.*
• *My goal is to do activities with others.*

If you are struggling to find a body mindful goal, look at one of your body mindless goals—the ones that leave you feeling self-conscious, down, and unsure of yourself—and think about what you are *really* after. What's driving your desire to accomplish that goal? Maybe you really want to look like your neighbor so you will feel a sense of belonging. Perhaps you want to look put together so you will feel respected and confident. Reflecting on that aspect of your goal—*how you wish to feel on the inside versus the way you wish to appear*—could be extremely enlightening.

Give it a try. Fill in the blank: *I wish to feel* _____.

Find Intention in Your Motivation

Let's identify the spiritual benefit underlying your body mindful goal. For example, an individual who wishes to feel energetic might derive joy living a more active life. A person who now stands tall may embody a sense of confidence from within versus only when she receives a compliment on her clothing.

Notice how both examples of body mindful goals in the previous exercise (*My goal is to feel energetic* and *My goal is to stand tall and look people in the eye when I speak*) are not dependent on outside forces to help you feel better about yourself, and both also lead you to a state of joy and confidence in your body by helping you shift your perspective and ultimately the thoughts you think and the words you say to yourself. Virtues like joy, confidence, and trust are the surest path to living a self-affirming body mindful life. When we learn that our strength lies in our virtues and not the size of our jeans or how we compare to others, we become self-empowered beyond measure.

Getting back to your goal: What is the spiritual gift your goal can give to you? Appreciation? Freedom? Joy? Patience? Hope? Name yours.

Your answer to that question is your intention. *Sankalpa* is a Sanskrit term in yogic philosophy that means "intention" and refers to a heartfelt desire, a solemn vow, or a resolve to do something. Sankalpa, or an intention, is a powerful motivational tool for manifesting your heart's desire in your life. An intention is like a compass that guides your actions, your choices, and even your thoughts and words. Intentions are positive forces and potent starting points for improving your relationship with your body.

Here are a few examples of body mindful intentions:

- *My intention is to cultivate joy in my activities.*
- *My intention is to appreciate all that my body does for me.*
- *My intention is to connect with my vitality.*
- *My intention is to cultivate patience with myself as I build strength.*
- *My intention is to find the courage to try new things.*

EXERCISE: Set Your Body Mindful Intention

Find a page in your journal or some white space in this book to write down your body mindful intention. Write it big and bold. Draw, color, or paint it too, if you wish. What's most important is that you record your intention so you can come back to it throughout this process. Believe it or not, by writing down your intention you will also plant a most precious seed in your psyche and heart.

To harness the potential of your body mindful intention in your life, we will ask you to revisit it, as well as your body mindful goals, several times throughout this book. This repetition will help you keep these words in the forefront of your mind. The practice of recalling your intention and goals will also help to "wire in" this language and reinforce your heartfelt desire to redefine your relationship with your body.

From Listen to Learn

The exercises you completed in the Listen step have prepared you for the next step: Learn. Personal growth requires the most profound sort of learning, a learning that directly impacts your deepest held beliefs and your most ingrained habits. This personal work is usually uncharted territory, making it an uncomfortable and difficult process at times. After all, it's much easier to observe someone else making a change than to be the one in the middle of it.

One of the first feelings you might experience during this process is that of being out of control. This is a common reaction to have when we don't know what will be unlocked in the recesses of our minds. That is why we asked you to name all the influences on your thinking in this first step. Understanding who you are and why you are gives you a sense of control. From this place of stability, you are more prepared to learn. This is one of the first things that psychologists seek to establish in individuals healing a traumatic experience. Once a trauma survivor can identify a trigger(s), the previous "victim" is empowered and aware that they have the power to determine their reaction. Hopefully you gained some helpful (or even profound) insights that will lead you to an even greater level of awareness in the Learn step. Take a few moments in your journal to recap key reflections from *listening* to yourself.

Chapter Summary

1. Listen is the first step of the Butera Method of Personal Transformation.

2. This step is designed to help you identify where you are now in your relationship with your body so you can set a course forward to create meaningful and empowering changes.

3. Listening to our truth can be uncomfortable and can also lead to breakthroughs that put us on a life-changing path that's been waiting for us to travel all along.

4. Your body mindful baseline (your current relationship with your body) is a starting point and is influenced by a variety of factors.

5. Your body narrative holds a wealth of wisdom about how your relationship with your body affects all aspects of your life.

6. Body mindful goals use positive, uplifting language that supports your physical, psychological, and spiritual health.

7. *Sankalpa* is a term in yogic philosophy that means "intention" and refers to a heartfelt desire, a solemn vow, or a resolve to do something. An intention is like a compass that guides our actions, choices, thoughts, and words.

8. A body mindful intention connects you to the spiritual gift of your body mindful goal and, like an anchor, helps you hold steady as you redefine your relationship with your body.

Whereas this chapter focused on *listening* to identify your starting point and set body mindful goals and intentions, the next chapter focuses on your unique *learning* style and qualities. As you read further and work through more self-reflection exercises, remember to keep your body mindful goals and intention in the forefront of your mind.

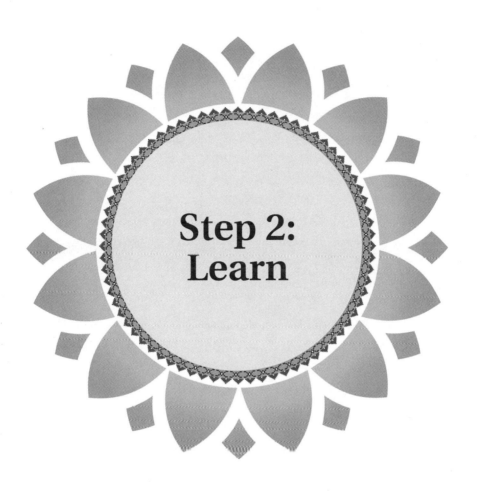

Step 2:
Learn

Now that you have an understanding of how your body narrative operates in your life and have established a starting point from which to grow, you can begin to pursue your body mindful goals and intention in the Learn step. *Learn* means to honor what you know and to invite new wisdom. First, we will take you through a series of exercises to discover how you learn and your unique qualities. Not only will this information be helpful in the upcoming Love and Live steps, but your insights from these exercises will function as your personal compass, for knowing how you wish to feel and how you learn is your unique pathway to inviting new wisdom into your relationship with your body. Next, we will take a deep dive into various social messages related to food, fitness, social media, and fashion and give you exercises for *learning* how certain words, expressions, and social messages influence your body image. You will study your self-talk and begin to identify body mindful language to bring into your life to support your body mindful goals and intention. The chapters for the Learn step will empower you to literally change your language and revise your body narrative.

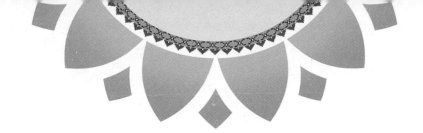

Chapter 4

Honor What You Know and Invite New Wisdom

"**S**ticks and stones may break my bones, but words can never hurt me!" This adage has been used to fend off bullies on the playground for over a century. First documented in 1862 in *The Christian Recorder*,[9] this saying is a powerful reminder that how we interpret and internalize our own and others' words affects the degree to which we "hurt." One major goal of this body mindful journey is to enable you to be free from how others' words and your own self-talk affect how you feel about yourself. For this step in the process, we need you to become aware of how you learn so you can unlearn a few things and then relearn how to listen to yourself. The exercises in this chapter will help you get in touch with your learning style and your unique nature. What does this information have to do with body image, you might ask? A whole lot, actually. Once we appreciate these aspects of ourselves, we can then use them to fulfill our body mindful goals and intention.

---

9. Gary Martin. *The Phrase Finder*. "Sticks and Stones May Break My Bones." https://www.phrases.org.uk/meanings/sticks-and-stones-may-break-my-bones.html.

Your Learning Style

Early memories are valuable sources for you to figure out how you learn. Our first memories may be shaped by photos, home movies, or stories told by our parents. How did you learn as a young child? What is the first thing you can consciously remember that you learned? Was it how to run? Sing? Color? Eat an apple? Play a game?

One of my (Bob's) memories was learning how to grab the lip of the kitchen sink as a four-year-old. I would put my left leg on the counter where it turned on an L shape and pop my right foot onto the countertop. Then I would roll my body onto the counter, and before anyone could see, I would pop onto the counter. Then, atop the counter, I could get a drink of water, pull cookies out of the cabinet, and simply feel like I towered over everything in the house. I am not sure why it was so much fun to touch the ceiling, but it was awesome for my four-year-old self.

There are many aspects of my personality bundled into that one memory: I learn best by doing; I move beyond preconceived limits when challenged; I try hard; and I am living proof of the idiom "Where there is a will, there is a way."

This memory reveals how I am willing to try things that seem impossible without giving up. It shows me that I like adventure and that I feel the work involved in achieving my goals is worth the effort.

EXERCISE: Getting to Know Your Unique Qualities and How You Learn

Write down a few of your pivotal memories and identify what qualities you possess. You might choose to identify a texture, taste, color, or smell related to a time in your life. You could also comment on the way you react to stories you've been told about your childhood, even if they're not actual memories you possess. Then use the information based on your memories or recollections to answer the following questions, jotting down your answers in your journal or right here in this book.

- How did you learn that activity?
- What basic traits helped you grow?

- What in your environment helped you learn?
- What was special about you (characteristics, talents, skills)?
- What situations help you thrive?
- Do you like to learn with others or by yourself?
- Are you more verbal or an observer or a reader?
- Do you like repetition, or is doing something once adequate?

Learning Weaknesses

I (Bob) was often impatient as a child. I was quick to learn things, and I felt trapped in situations where the teacher kept talking and didn't let us students try the activity. I felt like I was being tortured by drawn-out explanations that were incompatible with my learning style. Thus, I would then do my work too quickly and make errors caused by impatience, something I still do at times. The same traits that propelled me to ascend the countertop worked against me in other activities that were more cerebral. I also developed a fear of injury, because I would often be fearless at the start of an activity and end up with a cut or bruise due to that same impetuousness.

Examining your learning weaknesses is not about being good or bad, or right or wrong. Rather, it is an exercise in collecting more information about your nature and how you will handle other learning issues that we are about to tackle. By understanding your nature, you will get a clearer picture of the type of learner you are. In the chapters to come, you will learn how to put your learning strengths and weaknesses to work for you in lasting, body mindful ways. For now, reflect on your learning weaknesses in order to generate more wisdom about yourself.

EXERCISE: Exploring Personal Blocks to Learning

Grab your journal and write down some of your learning weaknesses. As a child, what were your stumbling blocks? What traits in your personality blocked your learning? When did you run from a challenge? What types of learning knocked down your confidence? Is there a hidden weakness in your confidence?

Your Nature Is Expansive and Unique

We are taught to introduce ourselves in short, succinct ways, like with our job titles, where we go/went to school, or where we're from. As a complex and multifaceted human being, your nature is much greater than a one-line description. Your abilities, preferences, talents, and disposition are ever evolving, making you an expansive and unique being. Your learning style is also a unique expression of one or some of these approaches:

- Heart person (leads with emotion; loving, giving)
- Spiritual person (seeks connection with oneself, others, and a higher power; big-picture person)
- Balance person (meditator, peacemaker)
- Efficient person (organized, disciplined)
- Energetic person (balancing all parts of oneself)

The next exercise invites you to realize your dynamic nature by expanding how you define yourself.

EXERCISE: Student of Life

Now that you have a sense of what kind of learner you are, use the following list to guide some self-reflection on the things that shape you as a student of life. We encourage you to take some time to reflect on all these self-defining points and explore how they apply to you specifically. Doing so will affirm your unique traits and qualities. It will also be a tangible reminder that your personal power is expansive and dynamic. You can make notes in your journal or right here in this book next to each line.

Personality Type
Personality
First awareness of your uniqueness
Strong traits
Weak traits
Introverted qualities
Extroverted qualities
Thinker or doer

Unique Identity
Personal goals
Priorities
Dreams, aspirations, bucket list

Unique Formative Experiences
Profound memorable experiences
Traumatic experiences
Special blessings or successes
Spiritual experiences

EXERCISE: The Story of Your Dynamic Nature

Take a few moments to review all the information you just learned about yourself. Sure, you probably knew most of this already, but perhaps you have never viewed yourself through all of these dimensions at one time or truly appreciated how dynamic you are—that you are much more than external identifiers such as your job title, where you live, the car you drive, or the size you wear. Pause and take in all the internal qualities that shape you and only you. Then spend a few minutes in your journal to give some narrative shape to who you are based on the Student of Life exercise. Tell the story of your dynamic nature without mentioning your body. This exercise is a wonderful reminder of how enlightening it can be to allow ourselves to own our qualities, traits, talents, blessings, hardships, and past experiences.

The Heart of the Matter

We are about to switch gears in a big way. But first, let's recap what you've accomplished so far. In the Listen chapter, you identified your body narrative and named your body mindful goals and a body mindful intention. Thus far in the Learn step, you honored what you know by taking a personal inventory of your learning style and your unique nature. The information you gathered about yourself up to this point will come in handy in the Love and Live steps. Your insights are also key to the material we are about to dive into, as *knowing how you wish to feel and*

how you learn best is your unique pathway to inviting new wisdom into your
relationship with your body and becoming a body mindful being.

Chapter Summary

1. Identifying your learning style and unique qualities is your personal pathway to inviting new wisdom into your relationship with your body.

2. Continue to notice your unique qualities and preferences as you learn in all areas of your life.

3. The insights you gain from identifying your learning style and learning blocks will serve you in many areas of life, including your relationship with your body.

4. By embracing yourself as a student of life, you allow your identity to center on your dynamic nature, unique gifts, and internal qualities.

This chapter bridges the gap between determining your starting point in the Listen step and exploring how language defines you in a series of upcoming chapters in the Learn step. After all, we inherit our language and its inherent underlying belief structures. Now it's your turn to define yourself and your body, and improve the world.

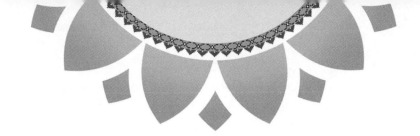

Chapter 5

Language We Live With: Slogans and Self-Talk

This chapter describes the complex and intricate layers of meaning that words have and their role in creating reality. We will share scientific research about the relationship between language and health and set the stage for you to examine your own language and body image in the four chapters that follow.

Intertwining Pathways of Meaning

Words give context to our experiences, dreams, and feelings. They also allow us to communicate and bond with others, giving us a sense of belonging to a larger group. Language gives us a means to organize our experiences and interactions. With words we can define, categorize, label, and rank. We know who we are by recognizing who we are not, which makes our ability to use words to define who we are even more important. Through words, we understand where and how we fit into our family, community, society, culture, country, and the world.

Words are merely steppingstones to endless and intertwining pathways of meaning, which we can explain only with more words. We think and communicate in words. Examining language typically isn't a priority for most people. Instead, we tend to use words without any critical thought as to what we are *actually* saying or how they impact us and others. For example, the person who over-apologizes walks through life saying "I'm sorry" multiple times a day for things that most likely are not worthy of an apology. The cumulative effect of all these apologies may leave that individual in a pervasive state of feeling wrong, bad, or not good enough. This person may also be overly concerned with pleasing others and gaining their approval. Simply repeating "I'm sorry" in this mindless way over and over will most certainly take a toll on the person's self-esteem and body image, because they will not feel confident to stand tall and steady in their body and life. Only the approval that comes from hearing "It's okay" or "You did nothing wrong" or "I'm not mad" or similar responses to the apology will provide a temporary boost in self-confidence. For the confidence to be lasting, however, it must arise from within.

Because we think in words, our thoughts are limited to the word combinations we know. Put another way, our thinking is bound by our language. Give a person new language through education and you expand their horizons. Show a person that language itself is a limitation and you gift them with the beginnings of enlightenment.

What Does Science Say about Language and the Brain?

The repetition of thoughts, behaviors, and patterns carve what are called *neural pathways* in our brains.[10] Simply put, with every repetition, these pathways grow deeper and deeper over time, making these thoughts, behaviors, and patterns our natural—and even habitual—reaction to people, places, and things that trigger the associated feelings. As such, it makes sense that it is hard work to change our relationship with our body, particularly if our typical reaction to our reflection is dissatisfaction. Our brain is used to traveling the dissatisfaction neural pathway in response to seeing our body. However, neuroplasticity is the brain's ability to reorganize itself and create new neural pathways. This

---

10. Christopher Bergland, "How Do Neuroplasticity and Neurogenesis Rewire Your Brain?" *Psychology Today*, February 6, 2017, https://www.psychologytoday.com/blog/the-athletes-way/201702/how-do-neuroplasticity-and-neurogenesis-rewire-your-brain.

means that with conscious practice engaging in new thoughts, behaviors, and patterns, we can literally rewire our brain. Repetitive practices like the ones you will learn about in the Love chapter lend a hand in this rewiring process. As you repetitively incorporate affirming language into your life, your brain will create new pathways, making this language accessible. A new variety of words will connect you with new thoughts and feelings that will hopefully move you closer to establishing an affirming relationship with your body.

Research has shown that our thoughts and feelings absolutely affect us on multiple levels.[11] Thoughts and feelings release neurotransmitters in the brain that directly affect our well-being, mood, and organs. In fact, according to many experts, our brain's structure and function can literally change just through our positive and negative self-talk.

The relationship between self-talk and performance is a popular focus of study in athletes. A study in the *Journal of Strength and Conditioning Research* evaluated the relationship between self-talk and performance in participants while doing a vertical jump test.[12] The researchers found that both instructional and motivational self-talk generated greater forces and higher jumps. Similarly, a systematic review of self-talk research concluded that athletes' performance benefited from positive, instructional, and motivational self-talk.[13] Negative self-talk didn't hinder performance, but it didn't help it either. This means that, at best, negative self-talk won't worsen athletic performance, but it also won't provide the performance boost that positive, motivational self-talk does.

11. Julia Scalise, "How Negative Self-Talk Sabotages Your Health & Happiness," *Brain-Speak*, December 15, 2016, http://brainspeak.com/how-negative-self-talk-sabotages-your-health-happiness.

12. David A. Tod, Rhys Thatcher, Michael R. McGuigan, and Joanne Thatcher, "Effects of Instructional and Motivational Self-Talk on the Vertical Jump," *Journal of Strength and Conditioning Research* 23, no. 1 (Jan. 2009): 196–202, https://www.ncbi.nlm.nih.gov/pubmed/19130644.

13. David Tod, James Hardy, and Emily Oliver, "Effects of Self-Talk: A Systematic Review," *Journal of Sport & Exercise Psychology* 33, no. 5 (Oct. 2011): 666–687, https://doi.org/10.1123/jsep.33.5.666.

These studies highlight the direct link between our thoughts (words) and our well-being, mood, and overall health.

If we consider multilingual nuances—the subtle differences in the meaning of words across different languages—we can also see how words influence our options for action, perspectives, and choices. For example, in the Western world, the term *yoga* means to do physical stretching and strengthening exercises on a mat. Similarly, in the West, Eastern martial arts are defined as physical combat or defense exercises. Yet travel east to the cultures of origin of these ancient arts and the meanings of these words are vastly different. Instead of describing types of exercise, these words refer to complete lifestyles.

I (Jennifer) encounter language nuances often, as my husband's family is Greek and they speak the language fluently. Whereas I say "turn off the light," my husband translates this from Greek to English as "close the light." This example is just one of many I encounter at home and at family events. Although these nuances in language do not cause a breakdown in communication, they do highlight cultural variations in meaning and how these variations influence a person's relationship to the world. In my world, the light turns on and off; in my husband's, the light opens and closes.

Slogans Are Powerful, and So Is Your Self-Talk

No words are original; rather, they are sound symbols passed down from generation to generation with various codes intact. These codes are powerful, and necessarily so, as the advancement of civilization depends on them. Slogans (short and striking or memorable phrases usually associated with advertising) and common expressions that circulate throughout cultures reinforce social ideas and values. These common and shared expressions live in the social consciousness and trickle into our own personal language in both blatant and subtle ways. We may even internalize the values expressed in some of these messages.

For example, take a moment to consider how many times a day or week you encounter language that claims you should feel guilt or even shame for "indulging" in a delicious dessert. We see this kind of language all over magazines, and it is the focus of entire articles and books. We hear it on TV and radio commercials, and we certainly can't miss it online or on social media. Entire industries exist for the purpose of cultivating guilt and shame around food. Now, think of how many people in your life speak the same or similar words. Before you know it, these outside social messages are forming and validating your internal thoughts. It's no wonder then that most of us feel obligated to say we "feel guilty" after eating dessert and we need to "work it off," or we believe that if we eat a certain food, do a certain workout, wear a certain brand, or post the perfect selfie, then we will finally fit in, be worthy, be beautiful, be thin enough, and be successful. The cumulative effect of these beliefs and others like them playing on repeat in our individual narratives and the collective consciousness diminishes our freedom to trust and accept our bodies.

Because we are tightly intertwined with the society in which we live, our work to redefine our relationship with our body must not exclude examining our relationship with the social messages we absorb, as they undoubtedly play a significant role in creating our body narratives. Over the next several chapters we will look at specific words and expressions that circulate throughout our social universe. We will examine four social facets (food, fitness, social media, and fashion), and a few well-known slogans or expressions associated with each one. The content included in these chapters is based on the results of our survey of two hundred men and women who were asked to identify words, expressions, and slogans used in various facets of our society that influence their body image.

You might find that some of the slogans in these chapters are relevant to you and others are not. We encourage you to focus on those that mean something specific to you, and work through the exercises at your own pace. The Body Mindful Journaling exercises at the end of each of the next four chapters will guide your self-reflection and can be used to practice responding in body mindful ways to language that incites feelings and emotions (both positive and negative) about your body and overall sense of self. This approach will do the following:

1. Expose flaws in social messages and thinking
2. Help you determine if and how certain language (your own and that of others) limits you
3. Empower you to rewrite disempowering words and thoughts
4. Give you practice being body mindful in your daily life

These chapters are designed for you to *learn* (honor what you know and invite new wisdom) through self-study or personal reflection how certain words, expressions, and social messages influence you. We recommend that you focus on the topics that are hot buttons for you, so you gain the most direct benefit from this process for your life. As we are discussing sensitive topics, we encourage you to reach out for support from trusted friends, family, clergy, or a therapist, should that be helpful to you.

Notice the Positives, Too

We understand that some of the material in the upcoming Learn chapters may push your buttons. It is meant to do this, so you can get to the root of some of the beliefs about your body that are causing you suffering. We also recognize that many positive, motivational slogans and expressions exist in our world as well, and we encourage you to include any of these that inspire you in the exercises and reflections that you do in this book. It's important to study your internal and physical responses to all language to gain insight into what kinds of words build you up, so you can include more of them in your daily dialogues with yourself and others. So please take the initiative to record positive slogans as well.

Why This Is Yoga

Although your experience of these next few chapters may feel different from that of the previous ones, in the true holistic spirit of yoga, our aim is to present you with a variety of experiences that will put you in touch with all aspects of your being—emotional, intellectual, energetic, and physical. These more social analysis–based chapters acknowledge that (1) we are not separate from the world, and (2) we respond to the world in numerous ways, all of which affect aspects of our being and life experiences, even if only subtly. By spending time with the world through the lens of language and body image, you will come out the other side more aware, more mindful, and more equipped to make meaningful changes in your relationship with your body.

Chapter Summary

1. Thoughts and feelings contribute to the quality of our lives, and words shape these thoughts and feelings.

2. Our words create our reality.

3. Language allows us to organize our experiences and interactions. With words we can define, categorize, label, and rank.

4. Through words, we understand where and how we fit into our family, community, society, culture, country, and the world.

5. Research has shown that our thoughts and feelings absolutely affect us on multiple levels and that positive self-talk alters performance.

6. How we interact with language can limit or free us.

7. Slogans and common expressions that circulate throughout cultures reinforce social ideas and values and can influence our body image positively or negatively, depending on how we internalize their meaning.

8. Our work to redefine our relationship with our body must include examining our relationship with the social messages we absorb, as they play a significant role in creating our body narratives.

9. Many positive, motivational slogans and expressions exist in our world, and we encourage you to include any that inspire you in the exercises and reflections that you do in this book.

10. To make this book work best for you, zero in on the topics in the next four chapters that are specific and relevant to your life.

In the next chapters of the Learn step, you will uncover how certain words and ideas that are prevalent in social messages influence your body image in concrete ways. From this learning, you will be prepared to take the step to rely on external validation less and define yourself from within more often. First up: social messages about food as a marker of morality.

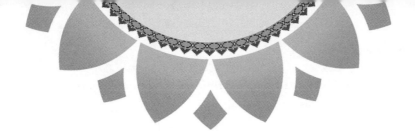

Chapter 6

Morality Language and Food

A common trend in social and cultural conversations is the labeling of food as good or bad. Linking this language and other morality words like them to food can lead us to believe we are good or bad based on what we eat. For some people, morality language may be inconsequential. For others, it can lead to feelings of guilt and shame. In this chapter we point out the ways morality language can potentially influence body image and self-worth. We also analyze a few well-known expressions and slogans related to food. Our goal is to make you aware of this language so you can learn if and how morality language affects your relationship with your body and begin to explore how you can incorporate body mindfulness into your own language and life.

To Eat It or Not to Eat It? That Is the Question

How many times a day do you bump up against this question (or one like it) in your mind as you navigate what, how, and when to eat? You are not alone if you experience moments of confusion or turmoil about nutrition, for we find ourselves embedded in a culture that complicates the definition of food and connects what we eat with our moral identity. Morality, by definition, is concerned with the principles of right and wrong behaviors and the goodness or badness of human character. Right and wrong, good and bad, and the many-layered meanings of these words have been applied to food, turning the act of nourishing our bodies into an issue of morality.

Before the refrigerator was invented for home use in 1913, families in traditional farming communities worked as a unit to cultivate nourishing crops. All hands were on deck. Men were generally responsible for field tasks such as animal care, plowing, harvesting crops, and using farm machinery. Women prepared and preserved food for the family and the livestock and maintained the farm compound. Children milked cows, weeded gardens, and harvested maple sap and berries for syrup.

The wisdom of the seasons dictated the family's diet. In the United States, for example, a bounty of snap beans, corn, cucumbers, melons, peppers, tomatoes, and squash were grown in the summer; pickles, carrots, root vegetables, and apples were enjoyed in autumn; garlic, leeks, onions, potatoes, and leafy greens filled the fields through winter; and herbs, broccoli, root vegetables, peas, cauliflower, and cabbage grew in winter for a spring arrival.

By its very form and function, the homestead encouraged and fostered eating. From the appetite-inducing hard work of farming to the natural rhythms of the seasons, a deeply intuitive intelligence was associated with food and hunger. Family members were raised to eat the food they farmed, so they never questioned which diet was the right one or when was the best time to eat. To be Pritikin, macrobiotic, vegetarian, or octovarian was not up for debate or even of concern; you were a farmatarian, and you ate what your culture and family ate. Choosing to have Italian, Mexican, or sushi for lunch was a decision that simply did not exist in the rural setting, and most likely neither did a preoccupation with the number of calories or grams of fat, sugar, or carbohydrates. In this way, traditional farming cultures represent a beautiful freedom and ease around food, eating, and hunger.

The Industrial Revolution, wartimes, and multiple other complex social, cultural, and political factors influenced the Western world's attitudes and values around food and led to what we are familiar with today. Rather than planting and harvesting in sync with the seasons, our social food norms are generally based on two values: speed and ease.

Within family or ethnic traditions, purposeful preparation of or celebration with food continues, even if sporadically. However, our daily experience is much less focused on food as an enriching source of connection with the land and community. Our day-to-day food choices are often dependent on the rituals we put in place to accommodate our lifestyle. Typically this means fitting in meals in the fastest and easiest way possible around work and family schedules. Without a foundation for preparing and sharing meals, we may lose touch with a natural or intuitive sense of how to feed ourselves, become reliant on diet fads, or get swept up in mixed messages about how, what, and when to eat.

Food Willpower

Many of the morality messages about food lean more toward convincing us that we are powerless—void of willpower—than powerful. If we buy into the "powerless" narrative, we can become overly tuned in to marketing messages and other sources that promote confusion, guilt, and shame around eating. As a result, we may become preoccupied with what the foods we choose say about our moral self-worth. From inherited food beliefs to marketing, from "fat" talk among friends and even strangers to "thinspiration" memes and images on social media, we are regularly exposed to messages insistent that the moral fiber of human character depends on "food willpower." The core message goes something like this: Depending on what and where we eat, we are either good or bad, disciplined or indulgent, virtuous or sinful, guiltless or greedy.

The more we rely on external validation to monitor our "goodness" or "badness," the less connected we are to our personal power, our inner knowing, and our appetite for food and all things in life. And the more we are attached to defining ourselves through words like *good* and *bad* or our perceived food "successes" and "failures," the less available we are to cultivate our dynamic nature and gifts. As you continue to read and work on the exercises in this chapter, you will learn how to shift away from the vice-and-virtue mindset to one based in personal empowerment.

Vice and Virtue

Like fashion trends, food groups go in and out of style. They are either revered as a virtue (behavior showing high moral standards) or demonized as a vice (immoral or wicked behavior). Instead of looking with anticipation at a plate of beautiful, colorful, nourishing food, we tend to see our food in terms of what it is *not*. From low carb to fat free, we are constantly reminded of what we are not eating. Such phrases are commonplace, and for many of us they signal safety, that we are "being good." These moral markers keep us pious eaters in a world of sinful food choices. Furthermore, actual food is swapped out for energy drinks, meal replacement shakes and bars, cleanses, and restrictive diets, all of which pledge to manage the natural rhythms of hunger to prevent a moral lapse.

In an era of "Nothing tastes as good as skinny feels," trends in clean eating and organic lifestyles hold the moral high ground, and in marketing terms, foods associated with these diets are virtuous. To eat "clean," for example, is to be "good," the implication being that foods not in the clean category are dirty or bad. We recognize that all food is not created equal, that quality of nutrition is essential for overall health, and that organic food is associated with health. We are purely concerned here with how the approach to moralizing food affects people's relationships with their bodies. For example, the repetition of hearing in our mind that we are bad or dirty because of what we eat can cause feelings ranging from self-doubt to self-loathing. Likewise, the repetition of feeling happy and healthful when we eat is uplifting and boosts our confidence. How does what you say to yourself about the food you eat influence your body image and self-esteem? Your answer to that question is what is so important for your own awareness.

An important point to consider that is outside the scope of this book is the question of how to navigate a food access network filled with hormones, fillers, and pesticides while maintaining a healthy relationship with food. In terms of physical health, this question is a vital one. For the purposes of *Body Mindful Yoga*, however, we are most interested in how morality language affects individuals' self-worth, and we hope that

the self-reflection exercises later is this chapter put you on a path to un-
covering this wisdom in your own life.

Real-Life Reactions

To learn firsthand how moral codes embedded in food culture affect
people's self-esteem, body image, and relationship with food, we sur-
veyed two hundred men and women ages eighteen and up. Their reactions to common buzzwords and slogans about food and diets illustrate
how internalized messages around morality and food may lead to confusion, guilt, and shame and strip us of our power to feel confident in
our food choices.

For example, "paleo," "gluten-free," "intermittent fasting," and names
of fad diets brought up a feeling in some of the survey respondents that
they were missing out or didn't belong if they didn't try these diets. These
words led others to express uncertainty about whether their current food
habits were the best choices. There was a sense of insecurity and anxiety
around whether they should continue their current practices (with which
they were content) or whether they should do what they perceived that
other people were doing.

Slogans related to thinness, like "Thin is in," "Get thin fast," and the
word "skinny," came up quite a bit in the survey responses. Some suggested that these words brought up in them a feeling of never being "in"
or good enough because they aren't thin or don't look like models in
ads. Others felt that these words and images of thinness alienate those
who are not thin, even if they are attractive, athletic, strong, and/or
fashionable, the overarching sentiment being that what matters most
when it comes to beauty is thinness.

Others shared that slogans that emphasize quick results are anxiety-
provoking. For example, phrases like "Get thin fast," "Improve your
body now," or "Remove flaws quickly" make people feel hyperconscious
and even worry obsessively about what's wrong with their bodies compared to ideal beauty standards. Similarly, the language used around extreme diets, such as "quick," "fast," or "You'll be better when...," were
also identified as overwhelming, making it harder for them to feel content with their bodies, lives, and simply the present moment.

Words like "cleanse," "clean," "organic," "detox," and "healthy" were tagged as terms that could be interpreted to imply that people's bodies are somehow dirty and need cleaning out. Others identified these words as indicators of morality, much like we've been discussing in this chapter.

Shame and guilt were also prevalent themes in the survey responses, as was anxiety around a perceived lack of willpower. For example, phrases like "fat free," "sugar free," or "no carbs" were described as reminders of what we are not eating, the implication being that it is more appropriate to focus on what we are not eating rather than what we are eating. Many expressed that this language suggests that guilt and shame are the appropriate responses to eating, versus enjoying a meal or nourishing our bodies for healthful reasons.

The story these comments tell is one of power—both the power of language and the power that we as individuals and as a society give away when we internalize moral codes around food and rely on these codes to validate or invalidate ourselves. The longer we remain in a body narrative with food that is based on morality, the more likely it is that we will relate to food as a reward or a punishment—two terms intricately tied to moral self-worth.

Food as a Reward and a Punishment

Considering the oversaturation of moral messages surrounding food in almost all facets of society, we can't blame our parents, extended family, or other people in our lives for experiencing food through the lens of morality. For example, in childhood, food may have been used as a reward and a punishment. From seemingly innocent statements like "Finish your homework and you can have a cookie" to more bribery-based assertions such as "I'll give you a cupcake if you stop screaming," the messages we receive can create unhealthy connections between behavior (or self) and food (the indicator of your moral goodness or badness). Similarly, using food to soothe or comfort a crying child (not including infants) teaches them to chew away feelings rather than share and work through them.

Consequently, now, as an adult or a parent yourself, you may continue to use food in similar ways with yourself and your children. We don't point this out to shame you, but rather to empower you through an awareness of this dynamic. Coming to this awareness on our own can be nearly impossible when the very same messages we absorbed in childhood are reinforced repeatedly within familial and social structures. Plus, it is not so easy to recognize inherited beliefs as faulty or unhelpful. After all, many of us have been taught that we deserve a treat when we are good and must do penance when we are bad.

Untangling Our Moral Worth from Food

If, as the moral code of food suggests, "you are what you eat," then it can be challenging to untangle your moral worth from the caloric value of the food you consume. Our goal in the pages that follow is to put you on course to take on this challenge in unique and body mindful ways. First, we will examine some of the slogans that have influenced the moral connotations and associations with food. If we study an idea from all angles and realize it's flawed, we can then let it go. By studying these slogans in this way, we wish to defuse the power they wield so that as you learn to be body mindful, you can reclaim your personal power through newfound wisdom.

The Body Mindful Journaling exercise at the end of this chapter will help you uncover how certain food slogans and related language influence your body image and self-esteem. You may be surprised by how little or how much these slogans impact you. Remember, these expressions are filtered throughout our society in a variety of visible and invisible ways, so much so that initially you may feel desensitized to them. It's likely, however, that some, if not all, of these slogans will strike a chord and open the door for reflection about what's possible when you transform disempowering thoughts into empowering, body mindful ones.

We recognize that there are many positive and motivational messages around food and health in our world. Our goal here is not to discourage you from embracing them if they serve you in helpful ways. Please continue to honor them in your life. We only wish to draw attention to other trends in language on this topic.

Before moving on to the slogan section, take a few minutes to do this short exercise:

EXERCISE: Check In: How Do You Talk about Food?

Journal about the morality language you use or encounter around food. Have you noticed this language before now? How does morality language influence how you view certain foods and eating them? What morality food rules or code do you follow? Where did you learn these rules or this code? How do they influence your body image?

Common Slogans and Expressions Related to Food

Here we examine a few well-known expressions and slogans related to food. Our goal is to create an opportunity for you to study how you relate or react to certain words and ideas so you can discover if and how morality language influences your relationship with your body. Use the Body Mindful Journaling exercise at the end of the chapter for yogic self-study and to record your insights.

"Nothing Tastes as Good as Skinny Feels"

Meaning: This slogan promotes self-deprivation and hunger and equates being skinny with happiness. Eating is displaced by the social rewards that thinness promises.

Origin: World-famous model Kate Moss coined this slogan when she was asked in a 2009 interview with fashion magazine *Women's Wear Daily* if she lived by any mottos.[14] Valued in the modeling industry for her "waif-size" body, Moss's definition of "skinny" was as clear as her body size. Her response set off a media war of words from all sides, igniting protests from body-image and eating-disorder activists.

---

14. Jenn Selby, "Kate Moss in Quotes: 'Nothing Tastes as Good as Skinny Feels' and Other Career-Defining Statements from Fashion's Silent Supermodel," *The Independent*, January 15, 2014, http://www.independent.co.uk/news/people/news/kate-moss-in -quotes-nothing-tastes-as-good-as-skinny-feels-and-other-career-defining-statements -by-9061975.html.

Moss's motto and many others like it, such as "Hungry to bed, hungry to rise, makes a girl a smaller size," "Waking up thin is worth going to bed hungry," and the infamous Special K slogan "How much will you gain when you lose?" have become rallying cries for the "thinspo" (thinspiration) movement, a social media trend that thrives on images and motivational quotes that encourage weight loss at all costs, no matter how harmful it may be. This movement reveres thinness at all costs as the promised land of happiness. These slogans ultimately ask their believers to sacrifice their health and vitality in exchange for deprivation. They also capture the pressure individuals feel to embody ideals.

Food and body codes such as these highlight the massive confusion that arises from the belief that the shape of one's body determines happiness. Rather than finding solace in spiritual concepts as self-identifying methods that lead to lasting contentment, such messages trick us into believing our shape and size must be controlled for life to "taste" good.

Perhaps the slogans and related ideas we discussed here struck a chord with you in some way. Turn to the Body Mindful Journaling exercise at the end of this chapter to work through your reactions to these words and create new body mindful expressions that support your body mindful goals and intention. To give you an idea of what we mean, here are a few examples of possible body mindful transformational statements in response to "Nothing tastes as good as skinny feels" that shift the focus from body size to self-connection. Use any of these statements that resonate with you, and create your own as well, for your own words hold the most meaning and power for you.

EXAMPLES OF BODY MINDFUL STATEMENTS

I respect my hunger and fullness.
I take time to honor and process my emotions.
Food is a divine gift.
I value my body.
I deserve abundance.

"You Are What You Eat"

Meaning: A person's health, well-being, and self-worth can be measured by the food they eat.

Origin: In 1825 the French gastronome Jean Anthelme Brillat-Savarin wrote in *The Physiology of Taste: Or, Meditations on Transcendental Gastronomy,* "Dis-moi ce que tu manges, je te dirai ce que tu es." ("Tell me what you eat, and I will tell you what you are.")[15] As with our current-day rendition of this slogan, this expression can be interpreted multiple ways, some of which are rooted purely in science and nutrition and others that are associated with moral integrity.

From a science and nutrition perspective, "You are what you eat" usually means that if you eat healthful foods, you'll be healthy, and if you eat unhealthy foods, you'll be unhealthy. This definition is a landmine that raises questions around the meaning of "healthy" versus "unhealthy." Various nutritional scientists and adherents of natural diets use this slogan or concept to explain their reasoning for choosing "pure foods" according to a particular plan. Those who advocate cleansing diets and cleansing the body with herbal practices such as skin brushing, drinking enough water, and colon hydrotherapy adapted this slogan to be "You are what you eat and what you don't excrete."

In popular culture, a person's outward physical appearance is considered what they are. A person's outward appearance is measurable, noticeable, and well defined by cultural norms. In contrast, it is impossible to examine on sight how the psychological disposition of a person relates to who they are, let alone their spiritual aspects. The 1960s' natural health revolution, along with the focus on obesity, helped the "You are what you eat" slogan become an ethical one, making a person's diet an outward symbol of both their body and their moral worth. The line of thinking goes something like this: Eat fat, and you are fat *and* irresponsible or unworthy.

---

15. Jean Anthelme Brillat-Savarin, *The Physiology of Taste: Or, Meditations on Transcendental Gastronomy,* Dec. 1825.

Further exploration of this general concept links back to the founder of medicine, Hippocrates, who is commonly credited as saying "Let food be thy medicine and medicine be thy food." Hippocrates moved the view of disease away from the realm of superstition into that of lifestyle, arguing that it's our life habits that provoke imbalance and eventually disease. He considered diet, environmental factors, and living habits to be the true culprits of disease. Centuries later, the phrase as we know it, "You are what you eat," is a distillation of Hippocrates's belief that food has a profound effect on health. The modern problem with this quote is that moral food codes want us to revere its literal meaning and attribute our self-worth to something outside of our true selves. No matter how we define a human being, individuals cannot be reduced to a list of food groups.

If this slogan hits a nerve for you, we encourage you to do the Body Mindful Journaling exercise at the end of this chapter to study your reactions and create empowering language to help you shift your perspective and boost your body image.

To give you an idea of what we mean, here are a few examples of possible body mindful transformational statements for "You are what you eat" that shift the focus to gratitude for nutrition as a life force. Use any of our statements that strike you as helpful, and be empowered to create your own too.

EXAMPLES OF BODY MINDFUL STATEMENTS

Nutrition supports my health
My meals nourish my body, mind, and spirit.
I offer gratitude for my food.
Food sustains my life, and I deserve to live life to the fullest.

"Guilty Pleasure"

Meaning: A guilty pleasure is something we enjoy that is considered to be not good for us or is regarded as bad or sinful. We atone for partaking in the sinful thing through guilt and self-denial.

Origin: The joining of these two opposing terms, *guilt* and *pleasure*, hints at the human psyche's attraction to charged situations, sensations, and emotions. Think about it: how often do you follow a controversial news report of a crime or natural disaster that you find both awful and alluring? In that tension, your mind may find some sort of fascinating struggle to obsess over or learn from. This same tension is encoded in language around food and guilt.

Many foods are coded as tempting and sinful (a guilty pleasure, so to speak) in part because humans seem to feel alive when there is an internal struggle between abstinence and excess. For example, the prehistoric search for food or water had significantly more life-or-death consequences than our modern-day drive to the grocery store. Because obtaining our food is such a casual experience—no chase, no seeking out a hidden patch of berries, no fear of being killed by a wild beast while gathering a meal—we have no excitement around eating an apple because it is simply sitting in the fridge or nearby on the counter. We don't even have to pick it off the tree.

But if the apple is a forbidden fruit, now there is some intrigue to be had! Put that apple in the Garden of Eden and all of a sudden an otherwise "virtuous" or "healthy" food is transformed into a "guilty pleasure." The mental energy spent fighting off the urge to eat that apple or chocolate or ice cream or another stereotypical "forbidden" food generates just as much excitement in the mind as does the planning, dreaming, and quest for that sinful treat. This tension may be further enjoyed if a veil of secrecy is inserted, for you can further relish this tension if you hide it from others. You may feel bad or devious afterward, but luckily the food industry is ever ready to help you rebound (or do penance), with a hefty list of guilt-free foods, cleanses, and diet shakes from which to choose. It's only a matter of time, however, until denying yourself pleasure backfires, and the hunt for pleasure makes you feel guilty.

Perhaps you can relate to some or all this explanation. If so, use the Body Mindful Journaling exercise at the end of this chapter to help you redefine the word *pleasure* as a life-supporting activity versus a cause of guilt or shame. Here are a few examples of possible body mindful transformational statements in response to "guilty pleasure."

EXAMPLES OF BODY MINDFUL STATEMENTS

Food is a gift from nature.

I enjoy health-giving activities.

I am worthy, as are all beings.

I deserve to enjoy food.

Pleasure is a natural human experience.

"Diet"

Meaning: A "diet," also referred to as a "fad diet," is a regimen that controls a person's food intake, with the goal of changing the shape of one's body or health. "Diet" can also relate to nutritional plans for managing overall health and resolving or supporting health conditions such as diabetes or autoimmune conditions. For our purposes, diets refer to fad diets focused on weight loss, not nutritional plans for overall health.

Origin: The ancient Greeks are the source of many of our modern health ideals, including the association between weight and discipline. That uber-disciplined society of scholars, with Hippocrates at the helm, preached that diet was a way of remaining healthy, for food was regarded as medicine.

A contradiction that is not often acknowledged is that dieting and "diet faddism" is only a problem in times of wealth. Humans needed an excess of food to secure their survival before something akin to a modern-day diet was considered. In the olden days, this sort of thing was reserved only for those with sustained wealth.

Because we have nearly unlimited food choices and countless fad diets to try, modern people have become confused about what to eat or which fad diet to try next. This confusion is rooted in a trend of looking for a plan to follow versus observing and understanding our body's responses to foods. To reclaim our diet is to spend the time required to know ourselves. There is also a social pressure attached to diet that may be as old as humans dining together. We like to belong as people. If our friends are doing a fad diet, then we want to join them in the process so we feel included.

What some people don't realize is that whatever diet they eat, it is still a diet. The problem is that *diet* is a loaded word that has evolved to represent the highest moral values of our society: restraint, control, will-power, discipline, rule following, restriction, and more. It's a means of shedding weight and proving our ability to uphold these high moral standards through the size of our body or our devout effort to "fix" our body.

What does the word *diet* bring up for you? Even if it triggers the slightest of twinges inside, we would like you to take some time doing the Body Mindful Journaling exercise at the end of this chapter to work through these ideas in your own life and create empowering language to help you shift your perspective and boost your body image. To give you an idea of what we mean, here are a few examples of possible body mindful transformational statements for "diet" and expressions like it. Notice how our examples shift the focus to cultivating self-trust versus relying on external sources.

Examples of Body Mindful Statements

I trust my body.
I know best.
I am self-aware.
I embrace my appetite.
I am worthy.

"Eat Clean"

Meaning: "Clean eating" and "eat clean" refer to eating foods as close to their natural state as possible and with minimal preparation.

Origin: Clean eating originated in pretechnological times. Without refrigeration or other high-tech methods of food packaging and processing, everyone ate "clean," meaning the food was not tainted by pesticides and hormones, as these did not exist until the modern era. Returning to that era's food principles, then, is the pure definition of our current-day expression "clean eating." Foods that are in their most wholesome form and animal products that are grass-fed, free-roaming, and hormone-free are considered clean. Raw foods are especially clean. If pollution is in the air, rain, and soil, then the organic integrity of food can be compromised, making it difficult to truly eat "clean."

Aside from this rational definition of clean eating is the use of "clean" as a moral signifier. "Clean" is positioned as the opposite of "dirty" and breeds suspicion about foods not labeled clean. Words like "organic," "clean," and "green" have also been positioned as "healthy" fad diets for weight loss, returning us to the mentality of "You are what you eat."

If these and related buzzwords are bothersome to you for whatever reason, we ask that you spend time working out these feelings and reactions in the Body Mindful Journaling exercise at the end of this chapter. This will also give you an opportunity to try on new, affirming language.

To give you an idea of what we mean, here are a few examples of possible body mindful transformational statements in response to "eat clean" and expressions like it. Use any of our statements that feel right to you, and be empowered to create your own as well, for your own words hold the most meaning and power.

EXAMPLES OF BODY MINDFUL STATEMENTS

Food is neutral.
I make good decisions.
I know how to feed myself.
All food is a gift.

EXERCISE: Body Mindful Journaling

If any of the phrases and words discussed in this chapter brought something up for you for whatever reason, we ask that you spend time working out these feelings and reactions through journaling. This will also give you an opportunity to try on new, affirming language. Respond to these prompts to help process what's coming up for you:

- Body mindful goals (from chapter 3): _____
- Body mindful intention (from chapter 3): _____

- Slogan/expression (from this chapter): _____
- Translate this slogan/expression in your own words.
- How do you relate to this slogan/expression? What does it mean to you in your life?
- What is your physical reaction to the words? Consider sensations, posture, and gut reactions.
- How does the slogan/expression influence how you feel about your body? Consider guilt, shame, comparison, and other related feelings.
- Write out the disempowering qualities of this slogan/expression.
- Acknowledge any self-empowering aspects of the slogan/expression. Explain why they are self-empowering.
- Practice transforming this slogan/expression into body mindful expressions that are free of guilt, shame, comparison, or other disempowering language. Revisit your body mindful goals, intention, and other reflections from the Listen and Learn chapters for inspiration.

Chapter Summary

1. Words like *good* and *bad* have been attached to food and eating, turning the act of nourishing our bodies into an issue of morality.
2. Modern inventions altered eating habits, making ease and speed the priorities over community and connection.
3. Foods are marketed as a vice or a virtue.
4. The more you let go of external validation to track your food "goodness" or "badness," the more connected you will be to your natural appetite for food and all things in life.
5. By paying attention to how you use and respond to morality language around food, you can actively begin to revise the way you speak and think about food.
6. Becoming aware of the food trends that have affected your life can help you regain control. You can reclaim power when you

establish your own plan, rather than looking outside yourself for the answers.

7. As you continue to read and work on the exercises in this book, you will learn how to shift away from the vice-and-virtue mind-set to one based in empowerment.

8. Honor the positive language around food and eating that resonates with you in affirming ways.

9. When it comes to food and eating, choose language that supports your body mindful goals and intention.

10. Your words are a pathway to redefining your relationship with your body.

As you explore your relationship to food in the Body Mindful Journaling exercise in this chapter, notice how some triggers are more powerful than others. Remember, the journaling exercises in this book are for the yoga practice of self-study, where you can reflect on what you know and invite new wisdom into your life. As you become increasingly self-aware, you will gain new insights to make empowering changes in your life. The process continues in the next chapter, where you will concentrate on understanding your relationship to the combat language of fitness.

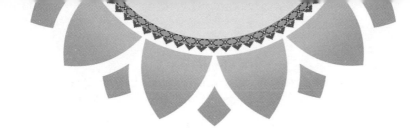

Chapter 7

Combat Language and Fitness

Motivational sayings about working out are highly beneficial for many people, inspiring them to make fitness a priority in their lives. Certainly we want to honor the value of motivational language for promoting healthy lifestyles. However, sometimes words and phrases that incite the spirit of combat are embedded in motivational fitness language, making the act of exercise about battling one's body. Our goal in this chapter is to highlight the theme of combat as it relates to fitness so you can learn if and how such language impacts your relationship with your body and your attitude toward exercise.

Fitness and Rivalry, Past and Present

Conquer. Fight. Beat. Eliminate. These words conjure up images of war, of armed opponents in pursuit of obliterating the other, and a fierce commitment to sacrifice and survival. They also characterize the spirit of competition: rivals competing to prove their athletic superiority and dominate the playing field. In both war and sport, only the fittest survive.

In ancient warrior societies, the most ruthless fighters lived to see another day, and their survival depended on the lethality of their bodies. By enduring rigorous physical and mental training in harsh conditions, bodies were transformed into weapons with which to conquer enemies. For example, in sixth-century-BCE Sparta, boys were bred to become elite soldiers as early as age seven.[16] They were subjected to harsh training and taught to take pride in pain and hardship, for such discipline was essential to navigate the rigors of warfare.

As is the case in modern-day militaries, extraordinary physical and mental fitness was of paramount importance. Spartan warriors were required to prove their physical prowess and proficiency in military activities and athletics, including boxing, swimming, wrestling, javelin throwing, and discus throwing. In this way, the well-trained, disciplined body of the soldier was a loaded weapon prepared to take out an enemy in battle or sport.

Although the current warfare landscape is drastically different from that of sixth-century Sparta, physical prowess remains a cornerstone of military culture. Modern athletic training bases its culture on warfare, which is not surprising considering that military training and athletics have been intertwined for millennia. Both employ boot camps, drills, interval training, weight training, sprints, long-distance running, and more to enhance physical and mental fitness, with the goal of defeating a foe or competitor. Attributes such as skill, speed, discipline, physical strength, mental toughness, self-sacrifice, loyalty, honor, integrity, and an uncompromising "win at all costs" attitude make a person a fit and worthy asset to the state or team, or both.

The Great Body Battle

Because fitness training has its roots in warfare and survival, current social and cultural messages about personal fitness for the non-soldier or noncompetitive athlete reverberate with themes of combat and threat. The language of warfare, complete with messages of self-sacrifice (like "No pain, no gain"), is overwhelmingly pervasive in the fitness industry. One need only scan the motivational workout memes on social media

---

16. Antonio Penadés, "Bred for Battle: Understanding Ancient Sparta's Military Machine," *National Geographic History*, Nov./Dec. 2016, http://www.nationalgeographic.com /archaeology-and-history/magazine/2016/11-12/sparta-military-greek-civilization.

or the headlines in fitness magazines to spot combat language. In the name of self-sacrifice, the seemingly highest ideal, we are beckoned to join the Great Body Battle: to fight fat, burn off flab, and turn soft flesh as hard as steel. We are sold the belief that, like warriors, we must do battle and push at all costs to tone and tighten, burn and shred, and eliminate bulges and bumps. From these messages we are taught that our bodies are the enemy.

The lengths we will go to get fit and feel validated, like "working out until I drop dead" or "pushing it to the limit," may seem like a small cost to pay when compared to the tradition of ancient warfare. However, personal fitness is not an act of war, and our body is not an opponent. Still, due to a desire to embody fitness in a world that can feel unforgiving to the unfit, many of us try to survive by containing, training, and shaping our bodies into an acceptable size. Even if that "ideal" size is reached, the inescapable language of warfare in fitness culture may leave us feeling uneasy and always on guard, for sometimes it can seem like we can't entirely trust that our bodies will not turn on us by gaining weight, turning soft, or failing us in some other way. Therefore, to be(come) fit is a personal battle reinforced by the social ideals that keep fitness tied to a militaristic mindset versus one based purely in health or enjoyment.

We recognize that there are many positive and motivational messages around fitness and health in our world. Our goal here is not to discourage you from embracing them if they serve you in helpful ways. Please continue to honor them in your life. We only wish to draw attention to other trends in language on this topic.

Armed for Battle

The warfare language embedded in fitness culture informs the going-to-battle attitude many of us bring to the gym, on a run, or even to a yoga class. Technology has upped the ante, literally arming us for battle. Wearable technology is a popular, growing trend. Forbes reported that the wearable technology market was predicted to exceed $4 billion in

2017. In 2015, just under 50 million wearable devices were shipped, and more than 125 million are predicted to ship in 2019.[17]

Certainly there is value in regarding physical fitness as a healthy lifestyle choice, and wearable technology may be a viable avenue for many people to accomplish this. Perhaps you, too, have found benefit from wearing a fitness tracker. We are not suggesting that using wearable technology is bad or wrong at all—we are not passing moral judgment on the devices or those who wear them. We only wish to point out the concern that these devices can take us outside of ourselves and lead us to become overly dependent on external criteria to determine how we feel about ourselves. For example, rather than focusing on how a workout feels or the enjoyment we experience, we might become consumed with monitoring ourselves like a piece of equipment or a machine. We can analyze acceleration, frequency, duration, intensity, patterns of movement, the number of steps taken, distance traveled, calories burned, and sleep quality. For some people this information may be very helpful, but for others it can lead to an unhealthy fixation. If low self-esteem, poor body image, and other psychological factors are involved, then this kind of tracking may lead to body comparison and feelings of guilt, shame, and even obsession with working out. No matter where you fall on this spectrum, what's most important is gaining an awareness of how fitness messages (and technology) influence your body image so you can empower yourself to make body mindful shifts in your life as you continue with this book and beyond.

In our survey of two hundred men and women, themes of angst, frustration, guilt, shame, and comparison showed up in almost all the responses we received about fitness. Several individuals commented on how seeing other people's before-and-after pictures of workouts and weight loss on social media brought up feelings of anger, jealousy, not working hard enough, and shame. People noted that the popular fitspo hashtags #fitandfab, #caloriecrushing, #fatburning, #burnoffthosecal-

---

17. Bernard Marr, "15 Noteworthy Facts about Wearables in 2016," *Forbes*, March 18, 2016, https://www.forbes.com/sites/bernardmarr/2016/03/18/15-mind-boggling-facts-about-wearables-in-2016.

ories, and others that focus on weight loss and fit body ideals made them feel like they must exercise hard every day, making it difficult to trust that they have permission to take rest days or exercise purely for the sake of being healthy.

Even fitness professionals shared that they feel similar pressures and worry whether their bodies will be viewed as good enough by potential clients as well as their peers. In fact, the word *fitness* was a point of contention, with many people expressing that it represents thinness and a sculpted body, rather than being a measure of health or even anything related to health.

Slogans like "Get thin and win" and "Strong is the new thin" were associated with pressure to have a certain body type for fear of being viewed as a loser. These kinds of slogans also brought up the pressure to be both thin and muscular, that being one or the other was not good enough. Some people expressed fear about being worthy or lovable if they did not match these beauty and fitness ideals. Others said that terms like "beach body" or "bikini body" make them feel like they don't deserve to spend a day on the beach if they don't have tight abs.

"Get fit," "Get lean," and "Lose weight" brought up a sense that they have to change their bodies to be a better person. Also, many shared that "No pain, no gain" made them feel like they have to take extreme measures to ensure they are working out correctly to lose weight or alter their body shape.

Several people expressed dismay around how the fitness world alienates individuals who are over sixty-five years old, with its emphasis on "strong, toned, and tanned," without concern for the needs of this age group, including cardiovascular, heart, and joint health. Similarly, language like "targets your belly fat," "lose your belly fat," and "burn belly fat" caused frustration for many respondents, making them feel self-conscious about an area of the body that naturally needs fat for biological and health reasons and ashamed of not having a flat stomach.

EXERCISE: Check In:
How Do You Talk about Fitness?

Do any of these survey comments resonate with you? Maybe you've thought some or all these things yourself, or perhaps you have a different perspective to offer. Feel free to jot down your ideas, thoughts, and feelings in your journal or here in this book. Then continue on to the next section on slogans, where you can study if and how fitness language impacts your body image. Your learning from these self-study exercises will open the door to new wisdom and help you redefine your relationship with your body.

Common Slogans and Expressions Related to Fitness

Let's examine a few well-known expressions and slogans related to fitness. Our goal here is to create an opportunity for you to study how you relate or react to certain words and ideas so you can determine how combat language influences your relationship with your body. Use the Body Mindful Journaling exercise at the end of the chapter to record your feelings and reactions and also brainstorm body mindful language to support your body mindful goals and intention.

"No Pain, No Gain"

Meaning: It is necessary to suffer or work hard to be successful.

Background: Thanks to Jane Fonda and her popular aerobics videos in the 1980s, "No pain, no gain" has become much more than a household phrase; it has become a social attitude and cultural mindset, a moral code of conduct and measure of a person's work ethic. Pain equals progress, and without pain, success counts less. Accomplishments are evaluated in terms of how much a body can withstand and a mind can endure.

"No pain, no gain" invokes a spectrum of desirable attributes that have become associated with the fitness, athletics, diet, beauty, and fashion cultures, from intensity, focus, and determination to sacrifice, self-denial, and punishment. Related slogans such as "Just do it" and "Beauty is pain" are intended to be motivational and inspirational and to push an individual toward a goal that is usually physical in nature.

Although these days "No pain, no gain" is associated with personal achievement, especially in the sports and fitness arenas, a form of the expression, "According to the pain is the gain" (which appeared at the beginning of the second century in *Pirkei Avot: Ethics of the Fathers*, part of didactic Jewish ethical literature), taught that spiritual gain is impossible without the pain involved in doing what God commands. The versions of this slogan that appeared in the 1500s and 1600s ring of the familiar modern connotation, which emphasizes that suffering is essential to progress and that hardship and achievement are inseparable. In his 1758 essay *The Way to Wealth*, Benjamin Franklin, in his persona of Poor Richard, stated, "There are no gains, without pains," to explain the maxim "God helps those who help themselves."

Ancient Greek thought may be at the root of many fitness slogans that have been reinterpreted in the modern era. All armies from the dawn of time would endure pain and show no sign of weakness to their enemies. Valor on the battlefield was meant to demonstrate not just the willingness to fight when the odds of survival were low, but to fight with courage and dignity. Hence, "No pain, no gain" was an attitude used in military training to prepare for the ultimate potential use of one's life for the sake of one's tribe.

The normalized cultural meanings of "No pain, no gain" can be internalized in different ways. For some of us, the slogan truly is motivational and even helpful. But for others, the message might lead to feelings of inadequacy or a need to push past healthy limits.

Even if commonly accepted phrases like "No pain, no gain" are popular, they may not be body- or life-affirming. How do you relate to this slogan in your own life? Use the Body Mindful Journaling exercise at the end of this chapter to work through your reactions to these words and explore new body mindful expressions that affirm your body and life. Here are a few examples of possible body mindful transformational statements in response to "No pain, no gain" and expressions like it. Notice how our statements shift the focus to cultivating balance throughout the body and in life in general. In your journaling, try out a variety of words and phrases that fit you best.

EXAMPLES OF BODY MINDFUL STATEMENTS

A balanced exercise routine supports a healthy body.
Moderation gives energy and strength.
Facing discomfort with love creates power.
Exercise increases my strength and boosts my energy.
I feel healthy when I work out.

"Survival of the Fittest"

Meaning: This is a biological concept related to natural selection that Charles Darwin popularized to explain why certain life forms thrive.

Background: Charles Darwin's writings on natural selection inspired biologist Herbert Spencer to coin the phrase "survival of the fittest" in 1864. Fitness as a biological concept refers to reproductive success within species.

Reproductive success is not the only reason for survival. Opportunity is another viable explanation. For example, if a species happens to endure in an unusual place, like underground or high in a tree, that species may survive during a climate-change event or natural disaster. After the disaster has passed, the adaptable life form may live on. Compared to most animals, humans are slow runners, swimmers, and climbers, yet our smarts and adaptability permit our survival. Perhaps the phrase should be revised to "survival of the crafty" or "survival of the adaptable." Humans are extraordinarily adaptable.

The words "fit" and "fittest" are typically used to describe physical attributes or body types. Images of ultra-fit men and women are often highly sexualized. Ironically, those who work out to extremes are at risk of elevated cortisol, which decreases the body's sex hormones (estrogen and testosterone) due to the strain on the body's systems and negatively affects fertility. On the other hand, inactivity also decreases fertility. In humans, moderate exercise is healthy for reproduction. However, fitness culture promotes extremes in its images and messaging, leading us to believe that we must exercise to exhaustion or jump on the latest fitness trend to "survive" *best*.

The word "fit" can also be problematic. The verb "to fit" has two meanings: (1) to be the right shape and size for, and (2) to fix or put (something) into place. In our number- and size-driven society (think weight, clothing size, calories, steps, miles, personal records, and so on and so forth), we are conditioned to "fit in" in all sorts of ways, from clothing styles to social groups to athletic teams. In this way, we consciously and subconsciously "fitness" ourselves to survive or "fit" the social expectations in which we live. Although many of us believe that "fit" can also mean ultimate health in body and mind, mainstream fitness cultural codes rarely portray a fit person to be one with a normal amount of body fat who takes time to relax.

What thoughts and feelings come up for you from this brief discussion about fitness as survival and vice versa? If "survival of the fittest" and other expressions like it stir up anything in you, we encourage you to do the Body Mindful Journaling exercise at the end of this chapter to work through your reactions and uncover what they mean.

Here are a few examples of possible body mindful transformational statements in response to "survival of the fittest" and phrases like it. Use any of our statements that resonate with you, and be empowered to create your own as well, for your own words hold the most meaning and power.

EXAMPLES OF BODY MINDFUL STATEMENTS
I am fit in mind, body, and spirit.
I strive to maintain balance in a changing world.
I flow between rest and effort.

"Win at All Costs"
Meaning: This expression means to put all efforts into pursuing and achieving a goal.

Background: The allure and glory of winning dates back to the original Olympic Games in Greece centuries ago and probably beyond. To "win at all costs" suggests doing so regardless of the expense, consequences, or casualties (figurative and sometimes literal). Exerting complete effort is the highest ideal in the pursuit of victory by individuals, groups, or teams. In a military survival setting, the army that exerts the greatest mental and physical effort may in fact be left to live. In this situation, winning equals living.

The drive to win at all costs is an endless cycle that can beget a greater and stronger drive to win. This attitude is most generally associated with athletes and sports teams, but we each have our own definition of what it means to win in our own lives. In other words, you don't have to be a professional athlete to be wrapped up in an identity defined by winning or losing. Winning can be associated with grades, personal relationships, money, sex, food, weight, fitness, business, politics, and much more.

To "win at all costs" can also drive personal competition with yourself by pursuing goals that may or may not be healthy, such as striving too hard to fit into a certain size, have a certain body type, or bench-press a certain weight. This drive to beat yourself again and again, to always outdo your last accomplishment, can also carry over into school, work, family, friendships, and other areas of your life. Since we live in a society that overvalues winning, perfection, and peak performance, to be average or good enough can feel like a failure, a loss instead of a win.

What internal reactions do words like "winning" and "losing" bring up for you? If these are hot-button words for you, we encourage you to use the Body Mindful Journaling exercise at the end of this chapter to work through your beliefs, thoughts, and feelings.

Here are a few examples of possible body mindful transformational statements in response to "win at all costs" that shift the focus from achievement to appreciating an experience. Use any of our statements that resonate with you, and create your own as well.

EXAMPLES OF BODY MINDFUL STATEMENTS
I give thanks for being able to play the game.
Challenges are a way to move my mind into the zone.

Learning from life is my victory.

I appreciate all my body does for me when I am active and when I am resting.

"Just Do It"

Meaning: "Just do it" means to seize the moment, to have the bravado to overcome fear or weakness and perform. This includes overcoming any feelings that are holding you back from moving forward with your life.

Background: "Just do it" is most popularly known as the slogan for Nike and is one of the core components of the company's brand.[18] What you may not know is that the inspiration for Nike's trademark slogan was the 1977 execution of Gary Gilmore, a convicted murderer whose last words before his death by firing squad were "Let's do it."[19] Gilmore's life and execution were the subject of the 1979 nonfiction novel *The Executioner's Song* by Norman Mailer, and the 1982 TV film based on the novel. "Let's do this" also made its way into mainstream sitcoms, including *Seinfeld*, *Roseanne*, and *NYPD Blue*.

"Just do it" remains heavily mainstream, as does the brand it represents. These three little words have become synonymous with "Go for it" and are found on posters, mugs, T-shirts, bags, keychains, stores, and gyms. Motivational images of this slogan abound on the internet and social media. With such a strong physical and digital presence, "Just do it" is embedded in the social consciousness, both inside and outside the fitness world.

Like the similar expression "Go for it," "Just do it" invokes a spirit of encouragement. Another similar one, "Go for broke," is a betting motto that implies one should literally risk everything for a win in gambling. Figuratively, this slogan means to risk it all to reach a goal.

18. Ryan Barrell, "Nike's 'Just Do It' Motto Was Inspired by Utah Murderer Gary Gilmore, Designer Reveals," The Huffington Post UK, March 20, 2015, http://www.huffington post.co.uk/2015/03/20/just-do-it-slogan-nike_n_6908946.html.

19. "Gary Gilmore Biography," Biography.com, Feb. 1, 2016. https://www.biography.com /people/gary-gilmore-11730320.

Speculation suggests that "Go for broke" may have its roots in the culture of the Wild West, when people traveled west during the California Gold Rush in the mid-1800s. Imagine an impoverished immigrant, or any person for that matter, achieving riches in their lifetime. To accomplish this would require tremendous faith, hard work, and risk taking. Perhaps there would even be a hint of exhilaration from time to time knowing that by "just doing it," by risking it all, a person might succeed. Narratives like this one—of immigrants arriving at the land of plenty or the underdog who overcomes the most difficult of trials and rises to the top—capture the essence of the very American attitude of "I can do it against all odds."

Like "No pain, no gain," however, this slogan can be internalized in different ways. For some of us, "Just do it" truly is motivational and even helpful in overcoming fear, trying something new, taking a risk, or confronting a challenge. For others, moments when "just doing it" isn't an option for whatever reason can lead to feelings of inadequacy, comparison, guilt, and shame. Others might also interpret this slogan as the pressure or obligation to exceed healthy limits.

How do you interpret "Just do it" in your life? What are the positive and negative connotations of this slogan for you, and how do they influence how you feel about your body and abilities? We ask that you spend some working out these feelings and reactions in the Body Mindful Journaling exercise at the end of this chapter. Doing so will put the power back in your hands to feel empowered in your body.

Here are a few examples of possible body mindful transformational statements in response to "Just do it" and expressions like it. Try creating your own too, for your own words hold the most meaning and power in your life.

EXAMPLES OF BODY MINDFUL STATEMENTS

I am capable.

The courageous honor their limits and act with wisdom.

The clever know when to ask for help.

It's okay to ask for support.

Giving my all includes honoring my body.

EXERCISE: Body Mindful Journaling

Which buzzwords and slogans around fitness and working out do you sense a reaction within yourself upon hearing or seeing them? We ask that you spend time working out these feelings and reactions through journaling. This will also give you an opportunity to gain insight into your relationship with your body and try on new, affirming language. Respond to the following prompts to help process what's coming up for you:

- Body mindful goals (from chapter 3): _____
- Body mindful intention (from chapter 3): _____
- Slogan/expression (from this chapter): _____
- Translate this slogan/expression in your own words.
- How do you relate to this slogan/expression? What does it mean to you in your life?
- What is your physical reaction to the words? Consider sensations, posture, and gut reactions.
- How does the slogan/expression influence how you feel about your body? Consider guilt, shame, comparison, and other related feelings.
- Write out the disempowering qualities of this slogan/expression.
- Acknowledge any self-empowering aspects of the slogan/expression. Explain why they are self-empowering.
- Practice transforming this slogan/expression into body mindful expressions that are free of guilt, shame, comparison, or other disempowering language. Revisit your body mindful goals, intention, and other reflections from the Listen and Learn chapters for inspiration.

Chapter Summary

1. Fitness training has its roots in military disciplines.
2. Motivational sayings around working out are highly beneficial for many people, inspiring them to make fitness a priority in their lives.

3. Oftentimes, motivational fitness language uses words and phrases that incite the spirit of combat, making exercise about battling the body or parts of the body perceived as wrong or unlikable.

4. The need for external validation may increase with fitness if your personal worth and happiness are overly dependent on your physical appearance.

5. Wearable technology can be helpful for monitoring fitness. Balancing your reliance on technology with an appreciation for your body and the healthful benefits of exercise is one way to live body mindfully.

6. Honor the positive language around fitness that resonates with you in empowering ways.

7. When it comes to fitness, choose language that supports your body mindful goals and intention from chapter 3.

8. By studying your reactions to messages about fitness, you will gain insight into how those ideas influence your relationship with your body.

This chapter taught you about the trend of combat language in fitness culture. Hopefully your own realizations about how this language influences your body narrative have been enlightening. Ultimately, the fitness movement is a wonderful thing for our generally sedentary society in which desk jobs are the norm and we spend an increasing amount of time sitting in front of a screen. Social media has us moving less and experiencing a type of communication that we will explore in the next chapter.

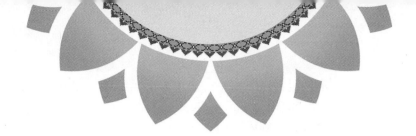

Chapter 8

Social Media and the
Language of Belonging

We live in a world where we are highly conscious of the presence of social media as a force for human interaction and connection. As you will learn in this chapter, social media taps into our basic human instinct to belong to the "tribe." This is one of the primary reasons that social media maintains such a prominent role in the lives of so many. After all, some people reading this book may not know life without the internet and social networks. Others can clearly remember the days without digital technology. Either way, social media is a powerful marker for self-study when it comes to how much we depend on external validation (or not) to determine our body image and self worth. Our goal in this chapter is to highlight the theme of belonging as it relates to social media so you can learn if and how the ways you use social media influence your relationship with your body.

What Does Social Media Have to Do with Survival?

It's nearly impossible *not* to have a relationship with social media, be it one of love, hate, or somewhere in between. Most of us are attached to the luxury of having instant access to Facebook, Twitter, Instagram, Snapchat, Pinterest, and other social media platforms. Our devices are loaded and ready to serve up a quick hit at a red light, give a lunch break update, or provide an evening's worth of amusement. And then there are the habitual checks throughout the day, like when we're waiting in line at the store or at the kids' bus stop or we're on a phone call or writing an email on a different device. Essentially, we could be on social media at any time of the day or night, at home or on the road.

At its essence, the virtual world of social media connects us to one of our most basic survival instincts: the instinct to belong. From the beginning of time, basic human needs were met in tribes, which consisted of families or communities connected by social, economic, religious, or ancestral ties. The tribe shared a common culture, dialect, and leader. Members worked together to gather food, maintain the home, and ensure one another's safety. The ways of life were preserved and reinforced by the tribe, with each member's role and existence dependent on their belonging to the whole group.

One Big Happy Personal Tribe

A major benefit of social media is that it links us to our personal tribes, and with every scroll through our newsfeed, we subconsciously seek to satisfy a deep desire to belong. These personal tribes are significantly more expansive and far-reaching than the tribes of old were. Platforms like Facebook and Instagram allow us to bond with friends and family all over the world. In the mere space of a post we watch babies grow up, teens go off to college, couples get married and divorced, and every life event in between. We follow what people eat, what they wear when they go to yoga class, and how many miles they ran. From the most mundane to the most significant events, we are privy to others' lives in intimate ways.

Not only does social media offer that comforting sense of "these are my people," but it also encourages us to make new friends and access other tribes or social groups. As we accumulate more friends that intersect with tribes removed from our personal one, our sense of belonging expands. Plus, beyond interacting with friends, we can join closed groups, create communities that support a cause, and network as professionals. We have instant access to current events and an outlet to voice our opinions. We can like and be liked—loved even. Every post is an opportunity to bond with our tribe, and every like, comment, share, and retweet reinforces our survival instinct to belong.

Social Media Literacy

Just as the survival instinct to belong has historically been reinforced through the tribe, so too have language and literacy been used to distinguish those who belong from those who do not. In ancient Roman society, for example, literacy was a distinct mark of the elite and clergy. Interestingly, medieval traveling drama troupes represented an early form of mass media. Performers spread social, cultural, political, and religious ideas of the day through plays and entertainment. These artistic groups existed in all sorts of forms and were easily hidden from censorship. The invention of the printing press in the 1400s initiated the education of a wider and wider audience. Although literacy was reserved for the elite, the masses slowly absorbed information through books and printed materials that were read aloud. This permitted the expression of ideas to slowly shift power in Western society away from the church to intellectuals and scientists. As recently as the late eighteenth century in England, however, women were discouraged to read novels for fear of them literally putting ideas in their heads. Women were to sit pretty and fulfill the roles appropriate to their class, not expand their creative and intellectual capital.

Social media is also a language, a form of literacy. Each platform speaks a similar but different language, requiring users to learn how to properly use it. This includes everything from understanding the interface to knowing what's a socially acceptable and appealing post. Depending on a person's "social media literacy"—meaning how well they use, read, interpret, and internalize what they encounter—these virtual worlds have the potential to reinforce social messages about which bodies belong and which do not. Therefore, despite social media's unique ability to cultivate a sense that we belong, how and what we use it for can also leave us feeling the exact opposite: not seen, not good enough, and not visually appealing.

On most social media platforms, the images in our posts are of paramount importance. Our sense of belonging is potentially strengthened or weakened depending on the attractiveness of the image posted. If it doesn't catch the eye, it's likely to be passed over without a like, comment, or share. So as we hold our phones in the palms of our hands and tally up our likes, we literally become outside observers of our bodies and lives. We study ourselves; we evaluate, judge, compare, self-surveil. We become an outside observer forever on guard about how much we belong or if we are following the rules of engagement correctly. And if we do, we are rewarded with likes, comments, shares, and retweets.

What Does Science Say about Social Media and Body Image?

A post that "underperforms" is probably no big deal for users who are moderately invested in social media. In contrast, more active, well-versed individuals who are possibly reliant on social media for a boost in self-esteem or are self-conscious about posting pictures of themselves may experience anxiety around rejection, increased body dissatisfaction, and decreased self-esteem. A 2010 study of 156 female high school students concluded that exposure to digital and print appearance-related materials on the internet was associated with both the internalization of thin ideals and weight dissatisfaction.[20] A 2013 study of 237 Hispanic girls aged 10 to 17 reported that peer competition and social media use were the strongest predictors of body dissatisfaction and lower life satisfaction.[21] More recent studies have found that girls between the ages of 10 and 15 who use social networking sites score significantly higher on preoccupation with body image than those who do not use social media. Participants in a 2015 study of self-proclaimed selfie users aged 19 to 22 reported that likes on social media improved

---

20. Marika Tiggemann and Jessica Miller, "The Internet and Adolescent Girls' Weight Satisfaction and Drive for Thinness," *Sex Roles* 63 (2010): 29–90, https://doi.org/10.1007/s11199-010-9789-z.

21. C. J. Ferguson, M. Muñoz, A. Garza, and M. Galindo, "Concurrent and Prospective Analyses of Peer, Television and Social Media Influences on Body Dissatisfaction, Eating Disorder Symptoms and Life Satisfaction in Adolescent Girls," *Journal of Youth and Adolescence* 43 (January 2014): 1–14, https://www.ncbi.nlm.nih.gov/pubmed/23344652.

their body image.[22] Most said they felt pressure to post compliment-worthy images. One significant conclusion of this study was that for this group of participants, posting selfies was more of an objectifying experience than an empowering one. A 2015 study of 800 men between 18 and 40 years of age found that men who were more likely to edit their selfies before posting them on social media scored higher in narcissism and self-objectification, which measured the degree to which participants prioritized their appearance.[23]

Certainly there are studies and anecdotal stories that demonstrate how social media is empowering. Still, the results of these studies and many others like them aren't necessarily unreasonable, especially given that social media is saturated with societal messages about beauty.

As a culture, we have internalized the media's ideals of beauty and personal and professional success. These ideals are reproduced and repeated on social media, which is partly why selfies have such an important place in social media literacy. Like the chief of the tribe who knew what its members needed to survive, the media has made billions of dollars assuming the same role, selling us the message that if we are tall, thin, toned, and tan, then not only will we belong, but we will also be valued for our willpower and perceived as confident and in control. Of course, the indisputable problem is that the media sells us ideals that do not ensure survival. Instead, we miss out on life, perhaps due to a fear of rejection or a preoccupation with body checking and comparing, which can play out as we strive to post visually appealing and attractive posts of our bodies. If we can package ourselves in ideal images, we may become celebrities within our tribe.

---

22. L. Rothery, "An Investigation into Young People's Experiences of Selfies in Relation to Self-Esteem and Body Image" (unpublished undergraduate dissertation, Manchester Metropolitan University, 2015).

23. Jesse Fox and Margaret C. Rooney, "The Dark Triad and Trait Self-Objectification as Predictors of Men's Use and Self-Presentation Behaviors on Social Networking Sites," *Personality and Individual Differences* 76 (April 2015): 161–165, doi.org/10.1016/j.paid.2014.12.017.

Real-Life Responses to Social Media

We learned from the results of our survey that body comparison is a highly common reaction to social media exposure, with many respondents reporting that today's constant stream of images can trigger jealousy, sadness, shame, and discontent with who they are and what they look like. Filters and other image-enhancing tools have upped the game when it comes to presenting ourselves to the world as picture-perfect, leaving many feeling pressured to constantly look ready for an image worthy of posting.

Others commented that the steady stream of so-called perfect bodies stirs up cycles of compare and despair, making it hard to feel self-assured and confident. Some shared that they have consciously chosen not to look at social media first thing in the morning, because doing so starts their day with negative self-talk about their bodies that ripples into a general overall feeling throughout the day of failure and not being good enough.

Some of our survey respondents talked about their desire to look like celebrities, from the size of their bodies to the length of their legs to their smiles and hair. Even though the respondents were fully aware that celebrities' bodies are usually Photoshopped, they still believed they needed to hold their bodies to the same standards, causing them to feel pressure to work out more and follow fad diets.

Do any of these sentiments about social media resonate with you? Maybe you've experienced similar reactions or feelings, or perhaps you have a different perspective to offer. Our goal in the next section and the Body Mindful Journaling exercise that follows is to encourage you to further reflect on how you relate to social media so you can get clear with yourself about which aspects of how you use social media empower you and which aspects disempower you. Our purpose is not to demonize social media or convince you to deactivate your accounts. After all, we all have a natural human desire to belong and feel connected to others, and social media is a wonderful tool for nurturing connections, especially if we can engage with our virtual realities with self-affirming language. Before jumping into the next section, let's spend a little time reflecting.

EXERCISE: Check In: How Do You Relate to Social Media?

Grab your journal and take a few minutes to reflect on these questions: (1) How does your basic human desire to be loved influence how you use and engage with social media? (2) How do you feel about yourself when you use and engage with social media? (3) What words do you say to yourself about yourself and the people you observe on social media?

Common Slogans and Trends Related to Social Media

Let's examine a few well-known slogans and trends related to social media. Our goal here is to create an opportunity for you to study how you relate and react to social media so you can discover if and how social media influences your relationship with your body. Use the Body Mindful Journaling exercise at the end of the chapter to record your feelings and reactions and brainstorm body mindful language to support your body mindful goals and intention.

Yoga Culture and Selfies

Meaning: "Yoga culture" is a modern term that refers to trends in the yoga boom in the West that began in the late 1990s and continues to this day. Yoga culture includes a focus on clothing and gear (mats, props, etc.), brands and trends, diet, related fitness practices, and "yoga selfies" on social media.

Background: One stereotype of both ancient and present-day yogis is that the practitioners were/are thin. This stereotype unravels, however, when we compare how yoga was and is practiced then and now. In contrast to the general modern-day understanding of yoga as a physical practice for fitness and stress reduction, the yoga of centuries ago was built on a range of ethical principles with the intention of ending suffering.

The originators of yoga were men who lived in ashrams or mountain schools over 5,000 years ago. The yogis dedicated their lives to practicing discipline over the body and mind. One such discipline related to diet, as fasting was a part of overcoming the physical plan to have a clear mind leading to spiritual enlightenment. This ascetic approach to the body as an unimportant tool for the spirit caused most monks to eat sparingly and to live utterly simply. (Please note that we are not espousing an ascetic lifestyle or a restrictive diet. Rather, our goal here is merely to share a historical point of view.) The emphasis on physical mastery and performance of daily yoga poses in combination with asceticism contributed to the trim build we associate with the ancient yogis. The irony lies in the fact that the external appearance of the yogi had nothing to do with attractiveness or other worldly aspirations. Achieving the modern ideal of a long and lean body clashes with the ancient yogis' mission to overcome the body in the name of enlightenment.

Another misunderstanding associated with yoga culture is that a flexible and thin body equals proficiency in yoga. Magazine covers, social media, and books promote bendy, contorted, long, and lean women. The irony is that, of the 195 verses of Patanjali's *Yoga Sutras* (an ancient collection of yoga texts whose title translates to "Rules of Yoga"), only three describe yoga postures. The purpose of yoga is to achieve enlightenment, yet in our modern culture, the physical branch of yoga has morphed into a fitness craze. Naturally, then, yoga culture upholds common cultural and social ideals related to beauty. This external show of performance vanity has nothing to do with the ancient yogis' desire to circulate the body's energy and sublimate sexual energy and sensual attachments to pleasures. In fact, the modern view of yoga would be to heighten the same appetites that the ancient yogis had hoped to sublimate.

Real-Life Responses to Yoga Selfies

Based on the survey responses we received, the surge in yoga selfies and body-positive accounts have contributed to the body-image angst so many people frequently experience. In addition to yoga selfies, social media has become saturated with advertisements for yoga clothing brands, yoga YouTube videos, and other related yoga topics. Certainly there are individuals and groups that aim to respect the ancient roots and principles of yoga. Still, in the West, yoga has largely become a fad that in many ways reinforces social ideals about beauty, fitness, and success.

The overwhelming feedback we received in our survey is that mainstream representations of white, thin, bendy, fit, and even ripped yoga bodies on social media and in the media make many people feel that yoga is not accessible to them. Some people expressed shame about their larger bodies as well as anxiety about going to a public yoga class for fear of being judged or standing out. Others expressed how being a yoga teacher with a larger body can cause doubt and worry about being perceived as a fraud by students and other yoga teachers.

Several respondents commented that popular yoga clothing brands tend to favor thinness and are not accommodating to more shapely body types. And although many commented that there are yoga images on social media that are inspiring, these same people also found it difficult to avoid comparing their bodies to the models in the ads or their friends in selfies, causing them to go so far as to question whether their bodies are worthy of practicing yoga in the first place. Interestingly, so many who shared their anxieties about images in yoga culture also alluded to the belief that none of what is represented in the media is what yoga is truly about.

We encourage you to take some time to think about your internal reactions to yoga as it is presented on social media and in magazines. If you post selfies (and there's no shame in it if you do), think a little bit about your intentions for doing so. What aspects of your engagement with yoga on social media are empowering and which make you question your confidence and personal power?

We encourage you to use the Body Mindful Journaling exercise at the end of this chapter to work through what's coming up for you in this discussion and create empowering language to bring into your life. Here are a few examples of possible body mindful transformational statements in response to yoga culture and selfies. Notice how we shift the focus from visual images of others' bodies to comments about self-respect.

Examples of Body Mindful Statements

I celebrate my uniqueness.

I am valuable. I respect myself and my life.

I am a student of life.

Yoga is a practice of presence and acceptance.

My yoga poses are a form of personal expression.

Yoga is for everyone, including me.

"Beach Body" and *"Bikini-Ready Body"*

Meaning: "Bikini-ready" is a term used to rally women to firm up their bodies for the summertime in preparation to show off their arms, legs, torso, and pretty much their entire body, as a bikini is akin to wearing no more than undergarments.

Origin: In 1961 the weight-loss salon Slenderella International launched an entire summertime campaign around "bikini body."[24] The company's ads promised customers a "high firm bust—hand span waist—trim, firm hips—slender graceful legs—a Bikini body!" As sexual morals softened in the 1960s, what was considered immodest dress in an earlier age became the norm, making the bikini a symbol of feminine and sexual liberation. This movement lifted some of the taboo around sexuality as being "bad."

A serious consequence of today's beauty and thin ideals, however, is that only select body types are viewed as bikini-ready. Every spring, without fail, the fashion and fitness industries as well as the media and social media blast out beach-body messaging through ads, sales, contests, motivational quotes, and an overload of images of ideal bikini bodies. As a result, many girls and women are sent into a body-image frenzy, causing them to turn to fad diets and workouts and allow the pressure to dictate their right to a day in the sun in a swimsuit.

Do an internet search for the term "bikini body" and you will find thousands of entries, from the latest diet to the best-looking bikini

---

24. Sara Coughlin, "Where Did the 'Bikini Body' Concept Even Come From?" Refinery29, April 13, 2016, http://www.refinery29.com/2016/04/108221/bikini-body-image-lies.

clothing and the best foods to eat to have that bikini body. Movie stars promote all kinds of impractical diets, for their livelihood depends on reflecting social appearance ideals. While men are judged for their fitness, they generally are not victims of the same sort of shaming, even if they are a few pounds overweight. Men are considered hefty, tough, big, or packing some bulk. Nicknames for women who fall outside of the body ideal are not nearly as kind.

Luckily, today there are movements working to encourage men and women to own their bodies in empowering ways, and *Body Mindful Yoga* contributes to that cause. We hope that one day the truly enlightened and liberated person will permit beauty to translate into diversity.

What does this discussion bring up for you? How does bikini-body messaging trending on social media and across mainstream media influence your body image? We encourage you to do Body Mindful Journaling at the end of this chapter to discover what thoughts, beliefs, and emotions are truly driving your reaction to "bikini body" and related language.

Here are a few examples of possible body mindful transformational statements to use in response to "bikini body" and expressions like it.

EXAMPLES OF BODY MINDFUL STATEMENTS

My body is a temple.
My self-worth is found within.
I set the trends for my life.
My body is worthy.
I respect my personal values.
I choose to experience the present moment.

"Hallmark Holidays"

Meaning: This is a term used predominantly in the United States to describe a consumer holiday, meaning its purpose is commercial rather than being a time to commemorate a tradition or a historically significant event.

Origin: Scroll through a social media newsfeed on and around St. Patrick's Day, Mother's Day, Father's Day, Halloween, or Valentine's Day (just to name a few), and what comes up, post after post? Ads, family pictures, funny memes, and all types of creative ways of wishing others well on these holidays. Sure, it can be fun and harmless. However, if we take a step back and look at this trend on social media, in mainstream media, and from a consumerism standpoint, we may bump up against possible feelings of peer pressure and comparison, both of which can directly influence our self-esteem and body image.

Did you know that Hallmark sells 1.6 billion cards at Christmastime and 150 million at Valentine's Day?[25] The pressure to participate in a holiday in the "right" way can cause us to lose sight of our own values as we strive to align how we choose to celebrate a holiday with what we see in our newsfeeds.

This sort of "holiday enhancement" on social media and in mainstream media paints an ideal as it romanticizes celebration and togetherness. In more sinister ways, the peer pressure that surfaces during holidays is also about body image. Let's take the famous slogan "New Year, new you." This expression predictably appears every December and is used to convince us that who we are is lacking, that our careers aren't good enough, our wardrobes aren't current enough, our diets are incorrect, and our bodies need to be ten pounds lighter.

Not surprisingly, gym and yoga studio membership sign-ups skyrocket at this time, as do diet and fitness fads. This messaging stirs up a social frenzy, with everyone convinced that the worthiest New Year's resolution is to alter, modify, rearrange, renovate, or transform. Many feel shamed into believing that the "you" of last year is not good enough. A "new start" is needed, along with a new wardrobe, a new diet, and a new promise of happiness.

How does what you see and hear around the holidays influence your mood, energy, and health? How about your self-esteem and body im-

---

25. Ethan Wolff-Mann, "This Is How Much People Still Spend on Christmas Cards," *Money*, December 14, 2015, http://time.com/money/4148180/christmas-cards-spending-2015.

age? Take some time to sit with your answers. The Body Mindful Journaling exercise that follows will help you work through your reactions and create empowering language to shift your perspective and boost your body image. Here are a few examples of possible body mindful transformational statements in response to the representation of Hallmark holidays on social media. Use any of our statements that resonate, and be empowered to discover your own as well, for your own words hold the most meaning and power.

EXAMPLES OF BODY MINDFUL STATEMENTS

Expressions of love have many forms.

Kindness is my currency.

I care about you and me.

I am connected to a higher power.

I celebrate in ways that honor my body, mind, and spirit.

EXERCISE: Body Mindful Journaling

During our discussion of the phrases and words in this chapter, if anything felt familiar or brought up new insights for whatever reason, we ask that you spend time working out those feelings and reactions through journaling. This will also give you an opportunity to try on new, affirming language. Respond to these prompts to help process what's coming up for you:

- Body mindful goals (from chapter 3): _____ _____
- Body mindful intention (from chapter 3): _____ _____
- Slogan/expression (from this chapter): _____ _____
- Translate this slogan/expression in your own words.
- How do you relate to this slogan/expression? What does it mean to you in your life?
- What is your physical reaction to the words? Consider sensations, posture, and gut reactions.

- How does the slogan/expression influence how you feel about your body? Consider guilt, shame, comparison, and other related feelings.

- Write out the disempowering qualities of this slogan/expression.

- Acknowledge any self-empowering aspects of the slogan/expression. Explain why they are self-empowering.

- Practice transforming this slogan/expression into body mindful expressions that are free of guilt, shame, comparison, or other disempowering language. Revisit your body mindful goals, intention, and other reflections from the Listen and Learn chapters for inspiration.

Chapter Summary

1. Social media connects us to our primal and collective human need to belong. What was once the tribe or village is now an online format of like-minded friends.

2. In the past, each tribe had its own unique language codes. We liken this to the way close-knit groups of friends develop inside jokes or gestures. This kind of communication within a group provides its members with an extreme feeling of belonging. Our survival used to depend on these versions of communication when living in the wild.

3. When used in the true spirit of connection, social media is a wonderful tool to nurture our natural need for a sense of belonging.

4. According to research, increased levels of comparison and other versions of self-criticism increase as a result of social media use.

5. You can empower yourself by paying attention to which aspects of social media influence your relationship with your body in both positive and negative ways.

6. You can master the use of social media to bond with others in healthy ways and remember to log off in favor of live interactions or after a limited time in order to remain internally focused.

7. Honor the empowering aspects of social media in your life.

8. Recognize patterns in your social media use that are disempowering.

9. If social media influences your relationship with your body in disempowering ways, call on your body mindful goals and intention from chapter 3 to help direct positive changes in social media use.

10. As your awareness grows, social media's negative side effects can be replaced by positive and uplifting experiences.

Related to our need to belong to a group is our desire for status in that group. In the next chapter, we will consider the influence of fashion and status on our relationship with our body.

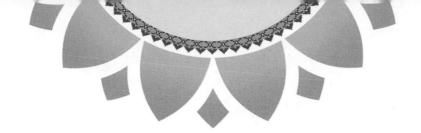

Chapter 9

Fashion and the Language of Status

As we discussed in the previous chapter on social media, one of our most basic human instincts is to belong. Cultivating connection with others is essential to our survival, for to live harmoniously with family, friends, peers, colleagues, our children, acquaintances, and strangers is fulfilling on many levels. Sometimes, however, the line between valuing connection and seeking approval can blur. Harmonious connection is both comforting and comfortable. Relationships based on approval—whether you are the seeker or the giver—are tricky because they are anchored in external validation. As such, approval-based relationships often lead to a rollercoaster of emotions that may include self-doubt, angst, despair, or a temporary high that lasts until the next approval-seeking encounter.

Now we turn our focus to the fashion industry and the theme of status, which has a strong potential to influence approval seeking among our peers and society in general. Our goal in this chapter is to highlight a few ways that status is emphasized in the fashion industry and give you an opportunity to determine if and how approval seeking may influence your body image and self-esteem in small or significant ways. Having an awareness of how this plays out in your own life will open the door to shaping an empowering, self-directed path versus one dependent on outside approval.

Rank and Style

Spend a moment with this quote by Diana Vreeland, the famous fashion editor for *Harper's Bazaar* (1936–1962) and *Vogue* (1962–1971):

> You gotta have style. It helps you get down the stairs. It helps you get up in the morning. It's a way of life. Without it, you're nobody. I'm not talking about lots of clothes.[26]

To be a nobody, to be insignificant, unseen, unheard—is there any greater fear? Ultimately, don't all our fears lead back to this single one? If we get super-honest with ourselves, most of us can trace even the most innocent and innocuous moments for approval, say from a teacher, coach, parent, or friend, to the fear of being perceived as unimportant or not good enough. Perhaps Ms. Vreeland's words weren't intended to be taken to such depths; nonetheless, her point captures a long-standing, centuries-old social belief: style, or fashion, is a visually powerful way to separate the somebodies from the nobodies.

Clothing as an indicator of rank and status is a historical phenomenon that developed to organize and maintain social hierarchies. For example, in China, a yellow robe was reserved for the emperor. In certain African communities, members of the ruling aristocracy wore large turbans and multilayered gowns made of expensive imported cloth. In Japan, the colors, weave, size, and stiffness of the kimono signaled social standing. Similarly, in thirteenth-century Europe, fashions were developed to establish and enforce social status. Dress determined one's economic status and social power, making fashion an effective way to control social class relations and maintain the social hierarchy. Laws were even created to align people's dress with their social class, and, as you can guess, the more affluent a person was, the more luxurious their

---

26. Lauren Alexis Fisher, "Diana Vreeland's Most Famous Quotes," *Harpers Bazaar*, July 29, 2014, http://www.harpersbazaar.com/culture/features/a2964/diana-vreeland-best-quotes.

clothing and appearance were. Although these laws were dismantled in Europe in the second half of the eighteenth century, notions of fashion as status persist in the present-day social consciousness, even if they manifest differently.[27]

The influence and confluence of various forces—namely mass production, class mobility, global capitalism, the internet, and social media—have contributed to the modern-day democratization of fashion, whereby all groups, even those on the periphery or those who are marginalized, have access to fashion, can imitate new styles, and can influence trends. Even still, messages and images circulated by the fashion industry can leave us feeling unsure of where we rank in our quest to adequately beautify our bodies. We need only flip through fashion magazines, scroll through #fashion on social media, or do some casual window shopping to internalize that, no matter how accessible and affordable style may be in the twenty-first century, the fashion industry, which includes the cosmetic industry, strongly values thinness and profits from our fears and inadequacies and our desire to "be somebody."

Like in days of old, when social class was enforced through dress, the fashion industry preserves this mentality through its models, mannequins, images, and language. The pressure to keep up with the fashions of the day, to fit into a certain size, and to wear certain brands can cause us to fall into negative thought patterns and use disempowering language about our personal status and bodies. Paradoxically, as we strive to empower ourselves by gaining status in the ways the fashion industry promotes, we may end up achieving the opposite result.

Clothing Sizes and Body Image

If you are prone to body dissatisfaction, no matter how slight or severe, the fashion industry can be challenging to navigate, especially considering a women's US size 0 (UK size 4) is the fashion industry's standard and falls drastically short of accommodating the average size of women

---

27. Katalin Medvedev, "Social Class and Clothing," LoveToKnow.com, http://fashion
-history.lovetoknow.com/fashion-history-eras/social-class-clothing.

in this country, which is a 16.[28] The standard clothing sizes we know today are significantly different from what they were fifty years ago. For example, a size 16 dress of the 1950s is comparable to a size 8 of today. Another staggering fact is that a size 8 in the 1950s would be smaller than today's size 0.

The shift in women's clothing sizes across the decades has been profound, and many women today can share stories of size inconsistencies between brands. Although clothing-size standards exist in the United States (but not in the United Kingdom), most companies do not use them. Companies dictate their own sizing, and although factors such as mass production and customer base purportedly play a role in determining sizes, the lack of consistency and sometimes large gaps in clothing size across brands and companies can add to the frustration and even anxiety we feel about shopping for clothes. It can also lead to or inflame low self-esteem and negative body image, fuel concerns about weight gain, and instigate unhelpful moral self-talk about food and exercise. Women might also box themselves in by shopping only at stores whose sizes make them feel that their bodies are "okay."

When we layer these dynamics onto any degree of body-image insecurity, the trying task of keeping up with trends and the pressure to imitate the Photoshopped models who embody "beautiful" can lead us further and further away from our ability to validate ourselves. As a result, we may become (hyper)focused on comparing ourselves to others and seeking approval in personal and material ways. For instance, some people might feel validated by another's compliment (which is only a problem if their security is entirely dependent on receiving the compliment in the first place), and others might rely on a brand or clothing size to boost their self-esteem, making the fall in self-regard a potentially steep one when these markers of status aren't achieved.

---

28. Diana Ngyuen, "A Brief History of Women's Clothing Sizes—and Why You Just Went Up a Size," E! Online, August 18, 2015, http://www.eonline.com/news/687475/a-brief-history-of-women-s-clothing-sizes-and-why-you-just-went-up-a-size.

Real-Life Responses to Fashion

In our survey, many people, especially women, expressed a range of feelings about how clothing sizes and body shapes are represented in fashion culture. People commented that it is rare to see an average-size woman in fashion ads, and if they are, they are labeled as such, making some feel that "average" and "curvy" models are used to pacify larger customers and persuade them to buy certain products. Others pointed out that larger sizes are carried only at designated stores, adding to the isolation that several people shared that they feel.

Many also referenced sizes 6 and 8 as the high end of acceptable sizes for women, the implication being that sizes beyond 8 are unacceptable or shameful. Along the same lines, several called out the lack of age diversity in ads, as well as the overt favoritism toward youth and young people.

Our respondents expressed frustration about the saturation of sexualized fashion ads, as these images and content reinforce the notion that women are valued for their bodies over their intelligence or meaningful contributions to the world.

What was most interesting and alarming to us about the survey responses we received was how common it was for feelings like anger, disappointment, or guilt to be followed up with a statement of comparison or even shame, accentuating how outside social forces can strongly influence our sense of self.

The Loneliness Loop

Even if you are content in your skin, brand-name comparison may drive a personal need for external validation. After all, there is some truth to the idea that we may dress to impress others. Associated with our instinct to belong are approval seeking and competition. We want to be valued by our peers; we do not want to feel lonely.

A study in the *Journal of Consumer Research* on the relationship between shopping and loneliness found that individuals who reported owning possessions as a measure of success and acquiring possessions as a source of happiness were associated with increases in loneliness.[29] This so-called "loneliness loop" of buying for status and/or happiness to alleviate loneliness is a self-perpetuating cycle that brings with it anxiety, depression, self-doubt, and low self-esteem.

Shopping addiction, which is a very real mental health disorder, can also stem from these states of mind. These more serious conditions may or may not be relevant to you, but nonetheless they highlight what's at stake when we invest our worth in status. We say this free of judgment and with the understanding that we are all surrounded by ideals, myths, and messages that idealize status.

EXERCISE: Check In: How Do You Relate to Fashion?

If you ever hear negative words in your head when you see fashion ads or stand in the dressing room or while shopping or getting dressed, we urge you to take time now do some journaling to learn about how your relationship with fashion (including the images, messages, ads, brands, etc.) empowers and/or disempowers you. What attitudes or mindsets do you have when you shop or get dressed for an event? Can you give yourself a compliment, or are you dependent on others to help you feel okay in an outfit?

Common Slogans and Trends Related to Fashion

Here we examine a few well-known slogans and expressions associated with fashion. Our goal is to create an opportunity for you to study how images and language about status influence your relationship with your body. Use the Body Mindful Journaling exercise at the end of the chapter to record your feelings and reactions and also brainstorm body mindful language to support your body mindful goals and intention.

"Life Isn't Perfect, But Your Outfit Can Be"

Meaning: Your outer appearance is a cover for your inner state of mind.

---

29. Rik Pieters, "Bidirectional Dynamics of Materialism and Loneliness: Not Just a Vicious Cycle," *Journal of Consumer Research* 40, no. 4 (December 2013): 615–661, https://www.jstor.org/stable/10.1086/671564.

Background: This slogan, whose author is unknown, appears in many fashion article headlines, is a popular marketing tagline, and circulates throughout social media, particularly Pinterest. You can find it on T-shirts, posters, wall décor, and many other items. At face value, it's a brilliant marketing strategy, as the slogan simultaneously speaks to the truth that life really isn't perfect and plays on most people's struggle to accept or be okay with their imperfections. Expressions that offer redemption for imperfection through clothing or other physical appearance–based solutions, such as exercise, dieting, and cosmetic surgery, can be problematic if they are internalized to mean that we must cover up or hide what we observe or label as imperfect.

This slogan also demonstrates how a thought pattern is code for myriad situations. Consider the ways this expression can be adapted to cover up any form of self-perceived imperfection in a variety of life situations, and the shame, guilt, and feelings of low self-esteem that might accompany it.

Life isn't perfect...

- but your friends can be.
- but your house can be.
- but your hair can be.
- but your kids can be.
- but your wedding can be.

This is an example of a thought pattern that tries to conceal internal feelings, thoughts, and emotions that surface when we encounter imperfection.

Let's take a quick critical look at the word "but" in this slogan. "But" is commonly used to contrast ideas and usually negates the first idea. Replacing "but" with linking words such as "and" and "because" creates a profound shift in perspective and attitude. For example:

Life isn't perfect *and* neither are you and me, so we can be ourselves and love despite our imperfections.

Or:

Life isn't perfect *because* everyone is unique; we are all uniquely lovable.

These statements have a much different feel than "Life isn't perfect, but your outfit can be." Simply changing "but" to "and" offers so much more freedom to be who we are in each moment, no matter what feelings we are experiencing. Even linking the two clauses of the original slogan with "and" instead of "but" opens the door to greater expression and authenticity. The sense of needing to cover up to put on a socially acceptable happy face dissipates.

How do you relate to this slogan in your own life? Do you feel pressure to hide certain feelings or cover up aspects of your life or body that are deemed imperfect? If this topic is relevant to you, we encourage you to use the Body Mindful Journaling exercise at the end of this chapter to reflect on what factors in your life may have influenced your beliefs about perfection and imperfection and presenting yourself to the world through a certain lens.

Here are a few examples of body mindful transformational statements in response to the slogan "Life isn't perfect, but your outfit can be." In the journaling exercise, you might try out language that shifts the focus from external identifiers to internal ones.

EXAMPLES OF BODY MINDFUL STATEMENTS

Life isn't perfect, but my loving and compassionate heart is.
Giving and receiving kindness is a true gift.
My gifts are unique and dynamic.
I let go of perfection.
I let go of competition.
I embrace all of me.

"There Are No Ugly Women, Only Lazy Ones"

Meaning: With money and effort, "ugly" can be fixed; therefore, women are lazy if they don't spend time and money to make themselves look better.

Background: Helena Rubinstein (1872–1965) was a business magnate who is credited for inventing the modern cosmetics industry.[30] She is remembered as a workaholic who adamantly believed that beauty could be attained through discipline and by buying her beauty products. Born in poverty in the Jewish quarter of Krakow, Poland, in 1872, Rubinstein's massive wealth and success represented the very ideals of discipline and effort that she sold to her customers.

One of Rubinstein's many famous quotes, "There are no ugly women, only lazy ones" is popularly used in fashion circles. This slogan ultimately asks, How far are you willing to go *not* to be perceived as lazy? It also asks, What are you willing to do to be beautiful? Like so many of the slogans we've discussed in this book, this language places pressure on individuals to constantly perform at high levels to achieve an image of confidence, control, and success—the opposite of lazy and ugly. We might go so far as to say that the fashion industry and other parts of society we've discussed in this book are in business because of our fear of being perceived as lazy, ugly, or fat.

Slogans and messages such as this one can lead us to believe that nothing we do is *enough*—we can't work out enough, eat right enough, dress well enough, spend enough money to improve our status, or work hard enough on our looks and at school, our job, home, and the gym. For those of us who have internalized this social message, which is so perfectly packaged in slogans such as Rubinstein's, we may experience degrees of guilt, shame, and comparison in certain areas of our lives. The very words "ugly" and "lazy" may bring up moral connotations, trigger varying degrees of body image concerns, and/or tap into a fear of failure and other work-ethic types of issues.

What does Rubinstein's quote bring up for you? What is your reaction to it, or how might you respond if you heard someone say this to a friend or even yourself? If there's even a slight stirring inside, turn to the Body Mindful Journaling exercise at the end of this chapter and explore

---

30. Cheryl Stonehouse, "Helena Rubinstein, the Penniless Refugee Who Built a Cosmetics Empire," *Daily Express*, March 16, 2013, http://www.express.co.uk/life-style/style/384696/Helena-Rubinstein-the-penniless-refugee-who-built-a-cosmetics empire.

your feelings about this slogan or related expressions in your own life. Here are a few examples of body mindful transformational statements in response to "There are no ugly women, only lazy ones" and expressions like it. Take time in your journaling to play with other words and phrases that resonate with you.

EXAMPLES OF BODY MINDFUL STATEMENTS

I seek beauty in the present moment.
All life is a beautiful expression of God's hand.
I am productive.
I spend my time in ways that honor my body, mind, and spirit.
My body is beautiful.

"Plus Size" and "Curvy"

Meaning: In the fashion industry, "plus size" refers to models who are a size 8 and up. Plus-size clothing typically begins at a size 16. "Curvy" refers to an hourglass body shape.

Background: "Plus size" and "curvy" are terms used to describe clothing, trends, and the size and shape of women's bodies. Today, the plus-size model, who until recently was considered a size 10 to 12, starts at a size 8, which is drastically smaller than the average American woman. The dictionary definition of plus size is "clothing or people of a size larger than the normal range." Considering that a plus-size model does not adequately represent a size larger than the normal range and also does not reflect the average size of women (size 16 in the US), this term is problematic. "Curvy" refers to an hourglass body shape. By this definition, body parts such as women's thighs, hips, bust, and waist are the focus, the key being that the waist size is smaller in proportion to the other parts.[31]

Both terms tend to be highly charged, as they call out and separate the perceived "lesser" body sizes from the "acceptable" ones. Individuals

---

31. Laura Beck, "Is This What a Plus-Size Model Should Look Like?" *Cosmopolitan*, January 11, 2014, http://www.cosmopolitan.com/celebrity/news/plus-sized-models.

with "larger" bodies are asked to shop at different stores or in sections dedicated to accommodating them. Some retailers only carry larger sizes online. Additionally, the existence of plus-size and curvy models suggest that these bodies are "other," "different," and even "wrong." Women who speak out online or in the media share that they feel marginalized and even discriminated against because of their size for these reasons.

If we go back in time a few centuries we find that "larger" female bodies were revered. For example, during the Italian Renaissance (1300–1600), a woman's body represented her husband's status. The full-figured woman (with full hips and a round stomach) was a symbol of her husband's wealth and proof that she was well taken care of. In Victorian England (1837–1901) and the Golden Era of Hollywood (late 1920s to 1960s), the hourglass figure was celebrated.[32] Body mindful individuals would hope to achieve awareness of all sizes as being neutral and of beauty as an expression of uniqueness. But we understand that it takes some work to get there, and we are here to help you begin this process.

No matter what your size is, take a moment and think about your reactions to the words "plus size" and "curvy." What do they represent for you? What feelings come up? What images show up in your mind? Turn to the Body Mindful Journaling exercise at the end of this chapter and work out your feelings about these terms and related expressions in your own life.

Here are a few examples of possible body mindful transformational statements in response to the words "plus size" and "curvy" that shift the focus to health-related comments. Use any of our statements that resonate with you, and be empowered to create your own as well, for your own words hold the most meaning and power.

---

32. Eugene Lee Yang, Mark Celestino, and Kari Koeppel, "Women's Ideal Body Types Throughout History," BuzzFeed, January 27, 2015, https://www.buzzfeed.com/eugeneyang/womens-ideal-body-types-throughout-history.

Examples of Body Mindful Statements

My breathing is strong.

I am vital.

I care for my body with healthy living practices.

I am always learning about health and wellness.

I embrace the wisdom of my body.

EXERCISE: Body Mindful Journaling

If any of the phrases and words discussed in this chapter brought something up for you for whatever reason, we ask that you spend time working out those feelings and reactions through journaling. This will also give you an opportunity to try on new, affirming language. Respond to these prompts to help process what's coming up for you:

- Body mindful goals (from chapter 3): _____
- Body mindful intention (from chapter 3): _____
- Slogan/expression (from this chapter): _____
- Translate this slogan/expression in your own words.
- How do you relate to this slogan/expression? What does it mean to you in your life?
- What is your physical reaction to the words? Consider sensations, posture, and gut reactions.
- How does the slogan/expression influence how you feel about your body? Consider guilt, shame, comparison, and other related feelings.
- Write out the disempowering qualities of this slogan/expression.
- Acknowledge any self-empowering aspects of the slogan/expression. Explain why they are self-empowering.
- Practice transforming this slogan/expression into body mindful expressions that are free of guilt, shame, comparison, or other disempowering language. Revisit your body mindful goals, intention, and other reflections from the Listen and Learn chapters for inspiration.

Chapter Summary

1. Although our modern society is more egalitarian, clothing choices and overall appearance are still valued indicators of rank, importance, and belonging.

2. External signals of status related to dress and appearance can lead to an externally powered sense of self-esteem versus the internal approach that body mindfulness encourages.

3. To be body mindful means to honor people of all sizes as whole, unique, and self-empowering individuals.

4. Making minor changes in your language choices can shift your current relationship to both fashion and your body from one that is limiting to one that is freeing. As you continue with the self-study journaling exercises, notice how making small changes in word choice has the potential to help you achieve greater, internally driven self-esteem.

5. If you redefine the role of fashion to cultivate body mindfulness, the superficial rules will remain in the history books but not take up space in your life.

6. Honor the empowering aspects of fashion in your life.

7. Recall your body mindful goals and intention from chapter 3 to help direct positive changes in your relationship with fashion and your body.

Over the past four chapters you have developed a powerful awareness of how language influences your relationship with your body. We covered major facets of society (food, fitness, social media, fashion), but there are many other social categories that we engage with daily. To demonstrate how you can investigate some other categories that are significant in your own life, we provide in the next chapter a template and examples for how to transform disempowering language into affirming, body mindful language.

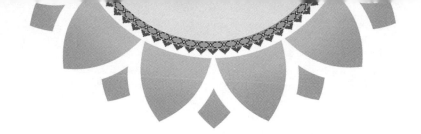

Chapter 10

Suggestions for Body Mindful Language in Your Life

Although we covered substantial ground in the slogan chapters on food, fitness, social media, and fashion, given that there are an estimated 25,000 idioms in the English language alone, we merely scratched the surface! Before we move on to the last two steps of the Butera Method of Personal Transformation (Love and Live), we are going to spend a little more time with the Learn step gleaning additional wisdom from language.

In this chapter, we expand our discussion to include religion, ageism, body part nicknames, and education/intellectual nicknames. We added these extra slogan categories to flesh out this process. However, you may apply the concepts and skills you have learned to any area of your life that impacts your body image or self-esteem. As in the previous chapters, we include suggestions to enrich your growing body mindful vocabulary. Our goal in this chapter is to continue to empower you to critically read and dissect language so you can shape your body image all the time, no matter where you are, with whom you are speaking, or with which aspect of society you are engaging. The insights you gain in this chapter will enlighten you to your ability to be affirming in areas of your life where language is binding you to a certain pattern of suffering.

The format for this chapter is simple. For each category, we

1. offer related assumptions,
2. discuss a potential body mindful perspective transformation, and
3. suggest body mindful statements.

Although this chapter is more of a summary than an exercise, we encourage you to spend time reflecting on buzzwords and expressions that cause even the slightest internal reaction, both negative and positive. You can work out your feelings about these slogans using the Body Mindful Journaling prompts from the previous chapters or create your own method for processing the information in this chapter. Some people like to journal, while others prefer drawing or collaging. Choose a format that works for you.

Body Mindful Review

Before we jump in, let's briefly revisit the principles of body mindful. When we are living body mindfully, we actively pay attention to the following:

1. How our desire to be loved by others (external validation) plays out in our relationship with our body—how we hold it, dress it, feed it, describe it, perceive it, and respect or disrespect it, and how we view others' bodies.
2. How our language either nurtures self-love in others or feeds their desire to be loved according to external ideals and messages.
3. Our relationship with our body is affirming when we rely on self-validation instead of external validation.

These body mindful principles enlighten us to the relationship between how we absorb and use language and how we feel in and about our bodies. So even words, phrases, and slogans that seemingly have nothing to do with body image actually might. Think about it: How do you hold your body when you feel confident? Sad? Angry? These examples are snapshots of the relationship between emotion (usually triggered by thoughts or words from ourselves or others) and body language, which is an indicator of body image in that moment. As you read through the following slogans and expressions, especially the ones that do not seem to be directly related to your body, pause and assess your body language. How does your body (including your face) respond to certain words or sayings? These physical responses are invitations to do some self-study and understand *why* this language influences your body image.

Religion

Assumptions

An entire book could be written about the influence of different religions on cultural thinking. The structure that religions provide to their believers is rooted in a time before the written word. As cultural containers of norms, rituals, faith, and security, religions hold immense psychic power. It's important to acknowledge that no two members of any religion sitting in the same house of worship interpret and internalize doctrines in the same way. How we take in or absorb a teaching in our own lives can directly influence how we experience our relationships, our bodies, and our place in the world.

Most world religions teach a mind-body split. Even in religions that espouse harmony between the mind, body and spirit, the spiritual and the material (the body) are often presented in opposition to each other. For example, the Spirit, or God, is presented in images and writings as flawless, pure, perfect, and omnipotent. In contrast, it is the weak human mind and the desire-ridden body that pull us away from purity and place us in a lowly mortal position. When interpreted this way, the Spirit is "good" and the body is "bad."

Although it is likely that no teachings say procreation is outright "bad," many do describe human desires as being less evolved than spiritual pursuits. The celibate monastics wrote about the pleasures of the flesh and the temptations of the body, establishing a paradigm that could potentially be internalized as "the body and its desires are bad." What follows is an opportunity for you to become aware of how you internalize the messages of your religious beliefs in relationship to your body. We acknowledge that this topic may be very charged, and we also want to make clear that we are not criticizing any religion or its teachings. Instead, and most importantly, we want to create a space for you to acknowledge disempowering interpretations with the intention of freeing yourself from those perspectives. We also acknowledge that there are positive teachings about the body in religions. Please take time to acknowledge or record those teachings for yourself, especially if they are sources of inspiration.

Body Mindful Perspective Transformation

We may transform the internalized belief that the body is bad and the Spirit good by developing a personal religious understanding that honors both the Spirit and the body. We can let go of the idea that the body is bad and instead practice moderation in all things. By being body mindful, you honor your body as a temple. Any negative view of a living being is, in and of itself, a nonspiritual perspective.

BODY MINDFUL STATEMENTS

I am a child of God.
My body is a temple for the Spirit.
My heart is glorious.
My body is a gift.
My spirit is joyful.
My body is a miracle.
My body creates.
My body is strong.
My body celebrates my spirit.
My spirit celebrates my body.

Ageism

Assumptions

As we've stated multiple times throughout this book, a central component of the body-image struggles many of us experience is related to the social and cultural definition of beauty as long and thin. "Youthful" can also be included in this definition. Expressions like "40 is the new 20" and "50 is the new 30" highlight our societal tendency to cling to a youthful identity. The medical and cosmetic industries make billions of dollars altering the human body. The beauty industry sells expensive products to rejuvenate skin, reduce wrinkles, cover up gray hair, and prolong a youthful appearance. Even health drinks with anti-aging benefits are promoted by the youthful-looking celebrities we adore.

Apparently, no one wants to be their actual age. A twelve-year-old wants to be sixteen and puts on makeup to look older. A twenty-five-year-old woman worries about her first wrinkle or gray hair. Older people may internalize the message that they no longer matter because their youth has faded. In turn, the young may internalize the belief that in order to matter they must make an effort to remain as youthful in appearance as possible, and middle-aged people might resist or be fearful of the natural aging process and struggle to feel at ease in their bodies. After all, we are hard-pressed to identify a beauty trend that encourages us to be ourselves at every age and not buy any body altering products!

Body Mindful Perspective Transformation

One powerful way to transform the belief that only youth matters is to appreciate the stages of life (birth, infancy, childhood, adolescence, adulthood, late adulthood, death) and honor the characteristics and traits these stages represent. This starts with the elders who may have fallen prey to anti-aging messaging. We need our elders to be elders and honor their age. In our modern age, we have mostly ended the apprentice model, whereby the blacksmith teaches the young blacksmith the trade, or the midwife (who is really your aunt) teaches you how to birth a child. In today's world there is no structure for elders to pass along their wisdom. A body mindful person needs to create their own forum to deliver wisdom in order to feel fulfilled as an adult. This may mean volunteering at a daycare center or going back to former places of employment to have lunch and listen to others. Essentially, you must find a way to pass down your knowledge.

We are going to bring up a word that is culturally taboo, and that is *death*. Our youth-fixated culture fears death. People are more likely to be content when they die if they feel that the wisdom of their life has been passed down. For example, the school teacher who mentors young college graduates and turns them into superstar mentors of children feels at ease when they retire because their career has gone full circle. We will not feel as old if aspects of our lives live on past our time. If we are not our ego, if we are not our body, if we are something more than both of those things, then we can feel connected to those who come after us. Therefore, it can be a blessing to honor the next generation by allowing them to be successful in their own ways. Doing so inspires an overwhelming sense of contentment in the older person, rather than sadness about getting old.

We need people to be empowered to be their true selves and be affirmed for being a kid or a teen or a fifty-year-old. Just be yourself and be proud of it. Honor others. Affirm others. Listen, accept, and love. This is body mindful living at its best.

BODY MINDFUL STATEMENTS

I affirm others.

I affirm myself.

I share wisdom by listening with love.

I identify with my divine self (not aches and pains or disease conditions).

I fulfill my duty with sincerity to my family, school, work, children, parents, church, and community.

I age as I am meant to.

I am wiser with each year.

As my body ages and changes, my ability to love others expands.

I am relevant; I matter.

My worth increases with age.

I am a valuable member of my family, school, work, church, and community.

My body is an expression of my life.

Body Part Nicknames

Assumptions

Hundreds of descriptive names exist for the eyes, nose, teeth, legs, feet, arms, ears, hips, stomach, and more. As kids, we are often given nicknames based on our physical features, usually the awkward or "imperfect" ones. Some of our childhood nicknames make us smile and others sting. We could ask you to mentally name a few parts of your body that cause you embarrassment or a few of your "imperfect" features that have been nicknamed by others (or yourself). You can probably name them very quickly. We know we can name ours!

Sometimes the labels we receive stick with us, making us self-conscious about our nicknamed imperfections. Or we might have been given nicknames based on positive qualities that we are also self-conscious about. Either way, if we've internalized these nicknames in certain ways, we can feel bad about certain body parts or features.

Body Mindful Perspective Transformation

One powerful way to release the hold of body part nicknames is to make your *uniqueness* your physical fashion statement. Every part of you is unique. Every part of every living thing is unique. If unique is in, then we all win, all the time, all day, all year, for the rest of our lives.

So let's go with this body mindful perspective: *Unique is in.* To help you internalize this new belief, we are going to define the archetypal power of a variety of body parts to cultivate body mindful self-awareness. See each part of your body as a divinely unique and amazing form serving you in your life.

BODY MINDFUL STATEMENTS

My head is shaped perfectly to hold my brilliant brain.

My ears are amazing capturers of sound waves.

My eyes present the outside world in 3-D color.

My nose is the world's best air filter, warming the air in winter and cooling it in summer.

My sense of smell could save your life.

My lips are tremendously sensitive.

My neck permits my head to move to and fro.

My tongue facilitates digestion, swallowing, and speech.

My smile and facial expressions communicate joy to the world.

My shoulders anchor my arms and sturdy my back.

My chest lifts as I breathe fully.

My belly protects my internal organs.

My core muscles keep my body erect.

My hips anchor my body.

My thighs give me power.

My knees provide adaptability.

My ankles spring me forward.

My feet connect me to the earth.

My legs and glutes represent my power and strength.

My body is wise.

Intellectual Nicknames

Assumptions

Our language is just as full of nicknames for the intellect as it is for body parts. Here's a short list off the top of our heads: Dumbo, Conehead, Numbskull, Airhead, Smarty Pants, Dork, Geek, Brainiac. You may also be familiar with Teacher's Pet, Brown Noser, Kiss-Up, Class Clown, and Show-Off. Although these nicknames are not directed at specific body parts, if they are internalized as hurtful comments, your self-image as a student could be affected.

Nicknames about our intellectual level, achievements, and pursuits can cause us to be overly confident as well as embarrassed. We might dumb down our intellectual image to fit in, or overcompensate in other areas of the educational experience, like athletics, to somehow make up for a "lacking" intellectual image. In both scenarios, we are adjusting our image to feel validated by peers. In the short term, this approach may work, giving us that comforting sense of fitting in. In the long term, however, being anyone other than ourselves becomes uncomfortable in all sorts of ways and jeopardizes our relationship with ourselves.

Body Mindful Perspective Transformation

We can cultivate body mindful awareness by recognizing the myriad ways we "fake" who we are, whether we are an intellectual or not. Any time we perform or act in ways that are not authentic, we disrupt our relationship with our being and body. Taking time to reflect on how denying or not honoring your abilities negatively impacts your self-esteem is excellent motivation for stepping into your personal power, owning your gifts, talents, and skills, and living a self-affirming life.

BODY MINDFUL STATEMENTS

My brain is a beautiful gift.

My smarts help me survive.

My ideas are unique.

My imagination is vivid and alive.

I am creative.

I am thoughtful.

I am considerate.

My brain is powerful.

Final Thoughts on Step 2 (Learn)

Our thoughts on these topics are far from final, to say the least. We could go through this same process of transforming body mindless assumptions into body mindful perspectives for dozens of categories and audiences, including parents, coaches, teachers, students, athletes, and professionals. Body mindful transformation would also be beneficial for individuals who struggle with anxiety, depression, eating disorders, trauma, and other mental health conditions. Considering that we all have a body and use language every day, body mindful self-awareness is truly a life skill we can all benefit from.

The last two steps of the Buteia Method of Personal Transformation, Love and Live, give you hands-on, real-life practice integrating the skill of body mindfulness into your inner life (the words you speak to yourself) and your outer life (your interactions with others). All the work you've done in the Listen and Learn steps will come to life in the Love and Live steps. With daily practice, your words and your body will align to create an affirming body image and life.

Chapter Summary

1. Continue to observe the areas in your life that are defined by others' views or various external circumstances. Pay close attention

to shifting your language in those areas so your energy goes toward raising yourself up versus pleasing others.

2. Notice any physical movements or postural changes in your body language when you use affirming language. These are powerful indicators and directly influence your body image in that particular moment.

3. Devise a simple way of memorizing positive "I am" or "My [X personal aspect] is good" statements so you can infuse your mind with new ways of succeeding in life.

4. By way of a refresher, the three principles of body mindful guide us to pay attention to the following:

   • How our desire to be loved by others (external validation) plays out in our relationship with our body—how we hold it, dress it, feed it, describe it, perceive it, and respect or disrespect it, and how we view others' bodies.

   • How our language either nurtures self-love in others or feeds their desire to be loved according to external ideals and messages.

   • How our relationship with our body is affirming when we rely on self-validation instead of external validation.

5. Body mindful self-awareness is a life skill that the next two steps of the Butera Method of Personal Transformation (Love and Live) will teach you how to integrate into your life and thus strengthen your relationship with your body.

6. To free yourself from disempowering attitudes, practice applying the steps of the perspective transformations we did in this chapter to pertinent areas of your life.

The Learn chapters have given you the chance to tune in to how you interact with the world through language. You have examined your internal responses to various prevalent messages in society and have spent time reflecting how certain words and expressions influence your body image. You have also begun to create body mindful language to bring into your life and interrupt the cycle of disempowering thoughts. Next, in the Love step of the Butera Method, you will discover how to integrate all this new wisdom into your life through a variety of yoga practices.

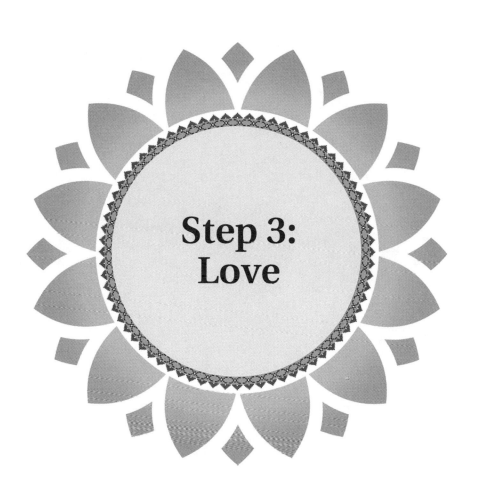

Step 3:
Love

In the Love step, you will learn how to use yoga to incorporate the new wisdom you gained from the Listen and Learn steps into your life. In the West, yoga is traditionally thought of as a physical or fitness activity. Yoga is vast in nature, however, and includes physical, mental, and spiritual practices that originated in ancient Indian philosophy. Yoga's philosophies offer guidelines for how to cultivate compassion and appreciation for ourselves (including our bodies), others, and the world. The Love step is an opportunity for you to incorporate body mindful yoga practices into your life that support you in creating an affirming relationship with your body. We've included a variety of mental, physical, auditory, and visual yoga practices to accommodate your learning preferences.

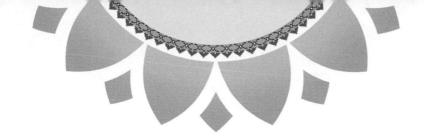

Chapter 11

Body Mindful Practices
for Your Inner Life

So far, you've been on an enlightening journey of self-study filled with courage and commitment to examine your relationship with your body. Working on ourselves in this way is not always easy or comfortable, and we encourage you to take the abundance of insights you've gained so far in the Listen and Learn steps and continue on your body mindful journey into the Love step. This step is all about converting wisdom into action. In other words, the Love step is like homework. It's an opportunity to practice what you've learned, test and integrate new ideas, challenge disempowering beliefs, and replace those beliefs with self affirming ones.

Because yoga has been the key to our own personal transformations and central to our professional lives, all the teachings and practices we share here are those we have experienced firsthand or practice regularly, meaning we practice what we preach! There's no doubt in our minds that without doing daily "homework," it is impossible to shift our body image in a positive direction. Such changes come only when we take responsibility for how we feel about ourselves and commit to daily practices that foster body mindfulness and boost our sense of self. The material in this chapter will help you establish an awareness of your inner dialogue and create daily practices as tools for incorporating body mindful language into your life, thereby leading you to a more affirming and empowering relationship with your body.

Tending to Our Inner Dialogue

The way we speak to ourselves in our own minds, even though no one else hears these thoughts, deserves tremendous attention. In yoga, the concept of *karma*—the notion that every action causes a reaction—is deeply rooted in the psyche. A personal insight starts the process of retraining the mind (action) through new emotional, mental, and behavioral patterns (reaction). There is no time frame that can be predicted before an insight becomes a habit and a new part of our identity. Each time you feel resistant to living your new insight is an opportunity to learn a new lesson. Each lesson learned is a gateway to feeling more empowered in your life.

Perhaps the first and most important lesson is to give yourself permission to believe it's okay to be who you are and where you are. Accept all of who and where you are in this very moment as you read these words. As soon as you accept that, the only thing left in your mind will be the peaceful feeling that acceptance leaves in its wake. Should you reject your thought or feeling as "bad," it will leave a wake related to the original problem. Your transformed thoughts need to be tended to with patience, compassion, and diligence. In time, your new insights will become a part of you in earnest.

Just as any skill we want to hone takes time, effort, and dedication to master, so too does this body mindful process. We don't just wake up one day and love ourselves more through pure willpower. Cultivating new body mindful language is wonderful, but it will make a difference only if we practice using it in our inner dialogue every day for the rest of our lives. We must challenge, rewire, and rewrite ingrained perspectives and beliefs, and that happens most fruitfully through dedication and repetition. We must build our mental endurance for this kind of personal work, and the exercises in the Love section serve as a great starting point for doing just that.

Your Inner Life

The Love step is concerned primarily with applying new wisdom to our *inner life*. Our inner life is who we are on the inside, independent of our social roles and identities. Although we play many roles in our lives, these identities do not represent our essential self, who we are on the inside. Our inner self is made up of our values, visions, passions, goals, and beliefs. It's where our virtues manifest and our unique qualities flourish.

Our inner life is independent of our outer appearance, but body-image concerns, when overly present, can overshadow the inner life, causing us to lose sight of our innate value and fall back into comparison or maybe even become swept up in guilt and shame. Therefore, living connected to our inner self requires a high level of self-awareness and dedication. Simply put, it takes daily practice. To support you in this effort, the Love step offers quiet, introspective rituals for you to practice body mindful language in your own mind and be proactive in creating a self-empowered body image.

Incorporating Body Mindful Action into Your Daily Life

So far, *Body Mindful Yoga* has included a combination of self-study exercises and wisdom points to help you break free from the bondage of words. In this chapter, we present you with a variety of yoga practices to incorporate into your daily life. A yoga exercise or practice is any activity that guides self-awareness. Some of the exercises we suggest are physical yoga poses, which are typically thought of as yoga in the Western world, and some tap into other dimensions of yoga, like intention and mantra. We've included a variety of mental, physical, auditory, and visual yoga practices to accommodate your learning preferences.

Recommendations

We strongly recommend that you make these exercises personal—just for you. Choose the practices that complement your learning style. Carve out a little time every day to devote to strengthening your inner dialogue and building your body mindful endurance. This is your time to take all you learned about yourself so far from this book and consciously chart new pathways in your life (and brain) by infusing it with new words, expressions, perspectives, and ultimately beliefs about your body and yourself. Following through with a consistent and active approach is a sure way to reshape your body image. These practices are the glue that makes it all begin to stick!

We also recommend setting time aside every day to do one or a combination of these exercises. Feel free to create a completely different exercise that's unique and suited to your learning style and preferences. If in the past you practiced a ritual that supported you in making a life change, we encourage you to incorporate that here. Make this exercise time 100 percent truly yours. This step empowers you to begin bringing it into your life so you can begin to feel real change within.

One more note: Notice how you talk to yourself when you do your practices. Notice the words that bubble up in your mind when you do yoga poses or meditate. Notice how it feels from day to day as you begin reciting body mindful words and expressions to yourself. Keep your journal handy so you can record your observations and insights. We ask you to notice these things not so you judge or criticize yourself or even overly celebrate your successes, but so you stay connected with your experience of this process, remembering that every observation is an opportunity to learn the next thing you need to know. This means noticing what feels okay, good, or terrible without judging yourself or giving up.

Recall Your Intention at the Start of Every Practice

First things first: revisit your body mindful intention from chapter 3. Sit quietly with it for a few minutes. Ask yourself if it still holds true or if it has changed since you first wrote it down. If it has changed, take a moment to formulate a new intention.

Now write your intention down again here or in your journal. At the start of each practice, revisit your intention. Say it to yourself a few times as a reminder of your heart's desire for your relationship with your body. Allow your words to motivate, guide, and inspire your experiences in these practices. As you grow, allow your intention to grow with you, meaning that if it shifts or changes, allow it to. Write down each iteration of your intention so you always have these body mindful words to come back to when you need them. It will also be fun in the future to track the evolution of your intentions.

Yoga Practices

Mantras, Affirmations, and Prayers

The word *affirmation* comes from the Latin *affirmare*, originally meaning "to make steady, strengthen." Since our spoken and unspoken words shape our reality, a key exercise for strengthening our body image is through the conscious repetition of positive statements in the form of mantras, affirmations, and prayers.

Mantras are words, sounds, or invocations that are used to aid concentration during meditation. Common examples are "Om," "love," or "peace." Affirmations are positive "I am" statements that can be used any time to cultivate positivity, such as "I am confident" or "I am strong." Prayer is an act of devotion and a way to ask one's higher power for help, comfort, support, and love.

Reciting mantras, affirmations, and prayers is a powerful way to integrate new ideas into your life. As is the case with exercise, when done consistently and with a tone of conviction, these high-vibrational thoughts can raise the levels of dopamine and serotonin, often referred to as our "happiness hormones." Therefore, positive words and slogans truly do help our minds feel better about our bodies and other areas of our lives that we may judge harshly.

EXERCISE: Body Mindful Mantras, Affirmations, and Prayers

Here are a few ways you can use mantras, affirmations, and prayer to inspire body mindfulness in your life:

- Pick a body mindful word or phrase from your journaling and spend a few minutes repeating it during meditation or in a less formal way (like upon waking up and going to sleep, before and after getting dressed, before and after meals, or in between tasks throughout the day), or set an alarm on your phone to remind you to repeat your word or phrase. You might also practice talking back to body mindless thoughts when they pop up by repeating your word or phrase to quiet down and replace these disempowering thoughts. An example is "unique" or "I am unique." Repeat this out loud or quietly to yourself for the duration of the exercise.

• Create visual anchors to remind you of your body mindful words. Write the words on sticky notes and hang them in places where you are sure to see them every day. Mirrors are an especially strategic spot to practice replacing criticism with kindness toward yourself. There's also something quite powerful about witnessing ourselves *choosing* to speak affirming language about our attributes. It may take time to become comfortable doing this, but it will be time well spent. Visual anchors will help keep you in practice.

• Bring your mantras, affirmations, prayers, or other inspiring words to life by painting or drawing them. Use your creation as a visual anchor and place it in a prominent area in your living space to remind you of the power of these words in your life.

• Create a vision board of elements that represent your body mindful intention. Vision boards are wonderful visualization tools that illustrate how we want to feel and what we want to bring forth in our lives. Get creative and colorful to tap into your fullest expression of your body mindful intention. Include pictures and words that inspire and motivate body mindfulness and connect you to your passions. You could also include activities and hobbies you want to try in the future. Design the vision board in any way you like, but be sure to include some body mindful language from your mantras, affirmations, or prayers.

• Create or purchase a journal dedicated solely to recording words and expressions that inspire body mindfulness.

• Choose a physical anchor, such as a beaded bracelet, a grounding stone, or another object you can wear or hold. Spend time daily repeating your mantra, affirmation, or prayer as you touch or carry your physical anchor.

Visual and Auditory Practices

Our senses of sight and hearing are nearly limitless in their ability to present us with new experiences that touch our lives in meaningful ways. Depending on your learning preferences, visual and auditory practices may be effective practices for integrating body mindfulness into your inner life.

EXERCISE: Body Mindful Visual and Auditory Practices

Try these body mindful visual and auditory practices. These exercises are less language-intensive and more sensory-focused.

- Spend time in nature appreciating the colors, sounds, creatures, and mysteries of the natural world. Practice watching yourself observe what you see and hear without judgment. In turn, observe your self-talk as it bubbles up, and practice matching the neutral observing you do of nature with that of yourself. For example, "I see a red bird" is a neutral observation statement. Through practicing neutral observation with nature, you can begin to practice it with yourself.

- View paintings, drawings, statues, and other pieces of artwork that inspire positive feelings. Notice the colors, textures, and other fine details that capture your attention. What unique qualities do you appreciate about these artistic pieces? If a work of art is especially pleasing to your eye, consider using it as a point of meditation. Gaze at it first thing in the morning for an allotted period of time as you recite your mantra, affirmation, or prayer.

- Watch or listen to lectures, presentations, movies, and plays with messages that reinforce a healthy mindset toward your body and self. Music also fits in nicely here. You can create a playlist of music that is uplifting and inspires self-confidence and empowerment.

• Body mindful–proof your environment. Fill your bedroom, office, and other living areas with items that support you in your body mindful mission. This means removing items that make you question your uniqueness, your worth, your body, and your confidence. Get rid of anything that makes you second-guess yourself. Choose to keep your space less filled up, or add colors, pieces of art, pictures, and other items that inspire positive inner talk.

Yoga Poses

The *asanas*, or yoga poses, make up just one branch of yoga. The other branches are guidelines for how to live a meaningful life and reduce suffering. They teach about moral and ethical conduct and how to attend to our health and nurture the spiritual aspects of our being. These philosophies teach nonviolence, moderation, truthfulness, contentment, nonattachment, and other concepts that support our inner lives.

The word asana means "comfortable seat." Traditionally, this definition of asana refers to how, with dedication and commitment, the physical poses teach us to concentrate, focus, and quiet our minds in preparation to "sit comfortably" in meditation. As a body mindful practice, we like to think of the definition of asana as learning how to sit comfortably in our bodies and listen to our true inner voice, so we can hear what we need to best serve our bodies, minds, others, and our world.

Yoga poses are a potent way to channel your body mindful efforts. As you hold the poses, breathe, and practice speaking to yourself in body mindful ways, you will literally rewire your brain and nervous system. Over time and with diligent practice, the kinder words will become more readily accessible, and the less kind words won't be as quick to show up.

Another profound benefit of practicing yoga poses is that they give you an opportunity to be embodied—to literally be in your body and discover news ways to relate to its parts as well as appreciate the whole.

Here we offer instructions for how to perform sixteen yoga poses. This set of poses will help bring balance to your body, as it targets all movements of the spine (side bending, forward folding, back bending, twisting) from a variety of orientations (standing, seated, supine, prone, inverted). We also list the attitudes or emotional qualities traditionally associated with each pose. This is not to suggest that poses are prescriptions for attaining a specific feeling, mood, or emotion. Rather, because the state of our body relates directly to the state of our mind, when done with intention, yoga poses can help us cultivate affirming thoughts as we grow stronger physically.

The yoga poses we suggest here are energizing, to foster feelings of empowerment. They also have an introspective quality to them that will allow you to tune in to your inner dialogue, study your self-talk, and test out new, self-affirming language. These poses can be done as a sequence, or you can focus on one or two poses at a time. After you familiarize yourself with how to do the poses, you can begin to incorporate them into your body mindful practice. If you are an experienced practitioner, we invite you to include other yoga poses that you know (and love) in these exercises. Feel free to get creative with variations, too.

Take time to set up your personal practice space and clear out any clutter, which includes eliminating distractions such as devices and other things that take you out of a state of focus. Include special books, pictures, and objects that are calming, grounding, and empowering. If you miss a day, it's okay No need to beat yourself up. Simply resolve to begin again, sooner rather than later!

EXERCISE: Yoga Poses

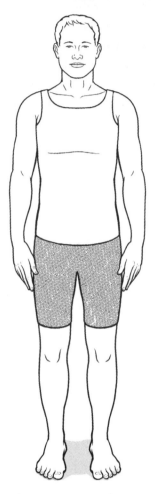

Tadasana (**Mountain Pose**)

Stand tall. Press your feet into the ground, especially the three points of each foot (the balls of the big and little toes and the heel). Stack your ankles, knees, hips, waist, shoulders, and ear lobes so everything is in alignment. Soften your shoulders, jaw, and eyes. Breathe with ease. As you stand tall and stable, connect to a sense of being sturdy, strong, and tall, like a mountain.

Attitudes: Strong, confident, grounded, steady

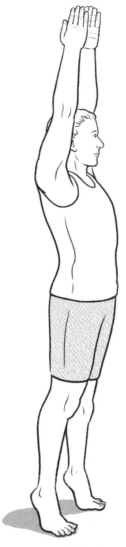

Talasana (Palm Tree Pose)

Begin in Mountain Pose. On an inhale, begin to raise your arms overhead as you roll your weight onto the balls of your feet. At the top of the inhale, you will have risen onto your tiptoes, with both arms above you. You can stand with arms parallel or with hands interlaced or in prayer position. Relax your shoulders. Hold this position for a comfortable length of time, then exhale and slowly lower your arms and heels.

Attitudes: Reaching to my fullest potential, faith

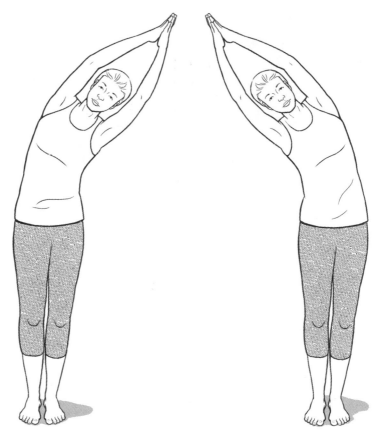

***Standing Ardha Chandrasana* (Standing Half Moon Pose)**
Starting in a standing position with your feet together, inhale and reach
your arms overhead. You can stand with arms parallel or with hands
interlaced or in prayer position. Exhale and lean your body to the right
while keeping your feet rooted in the floor and your top shoulder rolled
open. To increase the side bend, slide your hips to the left. Be sure to
press equally through both feet. Breathe with ease as you hold this position for a few rounds of breath. Inhale to center, then exhale to the
other side.

Attitudes: Fortitude, balance

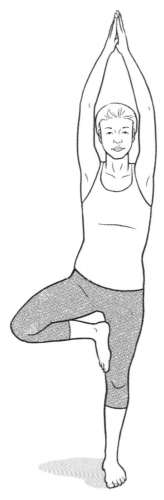

Vrksasana (Tree Pose)

Begin by standing tall. Root your left foot into the floor and plant the sole of your right foot on the side of your left leg above or below the knee but not against it. Keep your standing leg straight, but do not lock out your knee. Soften your eyes to a single point. Your palms may come together at heart center, your arms may open overhead into a V shape, or with arms overhead you can interlace your fingers and point your index fingers to the sky and cross thumbs. With soft eyes and relaxed shoulders, take several breaths and then switch sides.

Attitudes: Giving, rootedness, balance

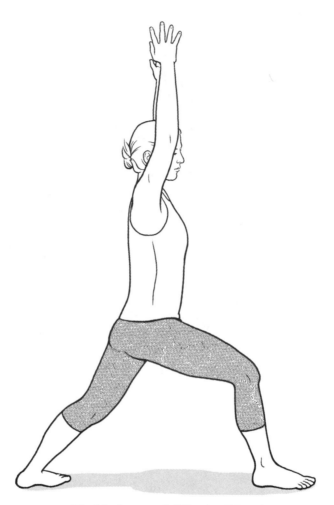

Virabhadrasana I (Warrior I Pose)

From Mountain Pose, inhale your arms over your head. Step your left foot back, turning your toes out and planting through the outer edge of the foot and toes. Bend your front (right) leg. Do not push the knee past the toes. Relax your eyes, jaw, and shoulders. Breathe with ease and the confidence of a warrior. Hold this pose for a few breaths and then repeat on the other side.

Attitudes: Perseverance, strength, open heart, forward-looking

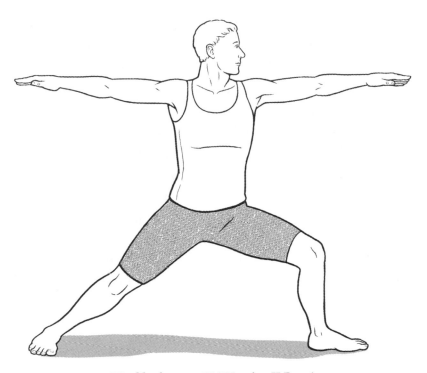

Virabhadrasana II (**Warrior II Pose**)

Step to face the long edge of the mat, standing wide-legged. Turn your front foot 90 degrees toward the front short edge of the mat, and turn the back foot to be parallel to the back of the mat. Inhale and lift your arms to a T shape so they are extended at shoulder height, pointing toward the front and back. Gaze steadily but softly past the front hand while your torso continues to face the long edge of the mat. On the exhale, bend your front knee toward your ankle. The knee can be over your ankle but not beyond it. Keep the torso and hips square while shifting the weight toward the front leg and foot and pressing into the outer edges of the feet. Remember to relax through your eyes, jaw, and shoulders. Hold this pose for a few breaths and then repeat on the other side.

Attitudes: Confidence, openness, strength, fearlessness

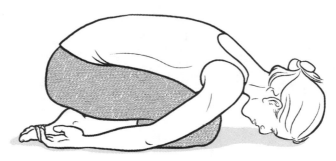

Balasana (**Child's Pose**)

Begin on your hands and knees. Bring your big toes to touching and sit back on your heels. Your knees can be close together or wide apart. Place your crown or forehead on the floor, keeping your seat on your heels. Extend your arms forward on the mat or rest your palms up beside your feet. You may open or close your eyes. Breathe with ease for several moments.

Attitudes: Humility, protective, nurturing

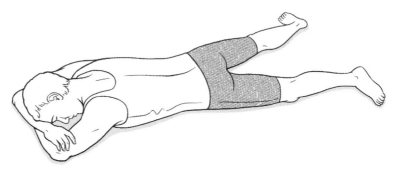

Makarasana (**Crocodile Pose**)

Lie face down with your forehead or a cheek resting on the back of your hands or folded arms. Bring your legs wide apart, with toes facing the outside. Notice the feedback from the floor as you breathe. Hold this pose for as long as you wish.

Attitudes: Supported, quiet, relaxed

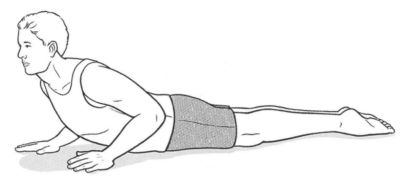

Bhujangasana (Cobra Pose)

Lie face down with your forehead on the mat, and place your palms under your shoulders. On an inhale, roll your forehead, nose, chin, and each vertebra off the mat to a comfortable height. Continue to gaze forward, not crunching through the neck. Draw your shoulders down and back. Bring strength into the lower belly and buttocks. Press into the tops of the feet and the pubic bone. Feel equal intensity in the lower and the upper back. If your breathing becomes short, strained, or irregular, or if your face begins to flush, it is best to come out of the pose immediately. Unroll through the chin, nose, and forehead, and rest your whole body on the floor, with feet wide apart and toes pointing outward. Rest your forehead or a cheek on the floor.

Attitudes: Transformation, achievement, forward-looking

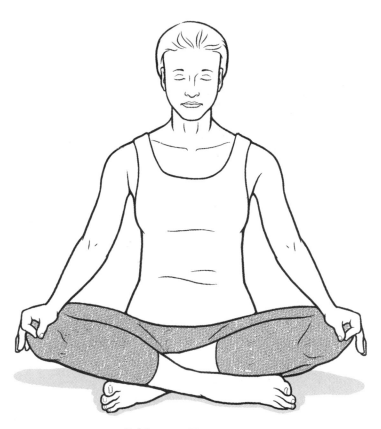

Sukhasana (Easy Pose)

Sit cross-legged, with your hands resting comfortably on your knees. Bring a slight smile to your face and tune in to your breath. Sit tall through your spine and bring relaxation to your toes, fingertips, shoulders, jaw, and eyes. Hold this pose for several deep breaths, taking time to reflect on what sensations you are feeling in your body, the quality of your thoughts, your emotional state, and your sense of connection.

Attitudes: Grounded, reaching for your true self, calm

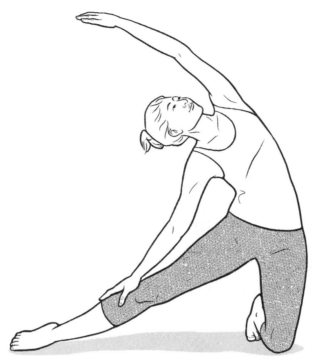

***Parighasana* (Gate Pose)**

Stand on your knees. For extra padding, kneel on a cushion or rolled mat. While the left hip remains directly above the left knee, extend your right leg to the right side, keeping your right hip, knee, and ankle aligned. Slide your right hand down the extended leg and raise your left arm overhead. Without tilting forward or back, side-bend over the extended leg. Inhale back to center and repeat the posture on the other side.

Attitudes: Openness to new ideas, possibilities, and experiences

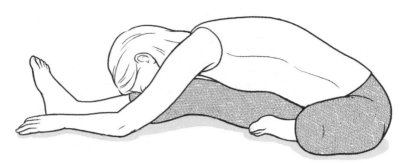

Ardha Paschimottanasana (Half Seated Forward Bend)

Begin seated, with both legs extended. Bend one knee to the side and place the sole of the foot against the opposite leg above the knee. Bring a slight bend to the extended leg. You may stay upright or fold forward to the degree that is comfortable for your body. Hold for a few breaths and then repeat on the other side.

Attitudes: Surrender, acceptance, faith

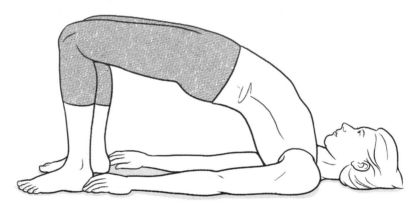

Setu Bandhasana (Bridge Pose)

Rest on your back and bend your knees, bringing them hip-width apart, with your feet planted close to your seat. Rest your arms long by your sides. Take care that your feet and knees remain in line with the hips throughout the entire pose rather than collapsing them in or out. Exhale and lift upward. Hold for a comfortable amount of time, breathing regularly and grounding into your legs and feet. Lower on an inhale. Repeat if you like.

Attitudes: Courage, relaxation

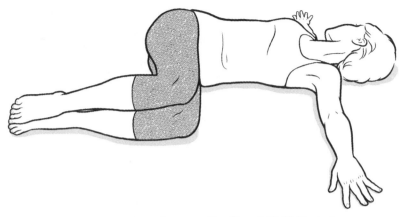

Supta Matsyendrasana (Reclined Half Twist)

Extend your arms to the side in a T position at shoulder height, and bring your knees in line with your waist. Exhale your legs to one side and ensure your feet are supported by the earth. If you are free of neck issues, turn your face gently in the opposite direction of your knees. Relax your jaw and eyes. You may close your eyes if that is comfortable. Breathe with ease for a few moments and then switch sides.

Attitudes: Surrender, wisdom

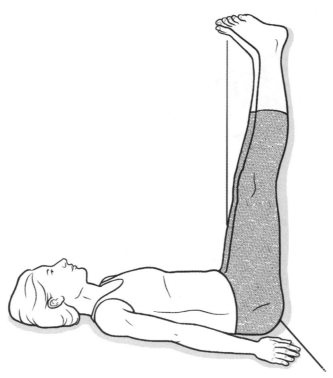

***Viparita Karani* (Inverted Action)**

Rest on your back, with legs supported by a wall and arms on the floor. Relax into the support of the floor and wall. Close your eyes if it is comfortable or gaze softly at your toes or above you. Follow your breath in and out, allowing the sound to soothe you. Hold this pose for as long as you like.

Attitudes: Relaxation, support, open to new perspectives, letting go

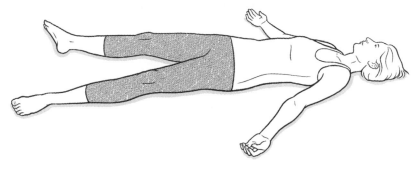

Savasana (**Corpse Pose**)

Lie on your back. Extend your legs long, with your feet as wide as your mat. Allow your feet to roll outward to create relaxation in the lower half of your body. Let your arms be long and away from your sides. Relax your hands and turn your palms up. If comfortable, close your eyes. Ask your entire body to rest and restore. Follow the natural rhythm of your breath, creating calm in your mind and balance in your body. Use this pose to fully rest. You can also repeat mantras and other body-affirming statements that you are practicing in your other yoga practices. Stay in the pose for as long as you like.

Attitudes: Relaxation, letting go, surrender, acceptance

EXERCISE: Body Mindful Yoga Pose Practices

Here are a few ways you can do yoga poses to support your body mindful practice:

- Repeat your body mindful intention to yourself as you hold a yoga pose or throughout a series of poses. Say it in your mind or out loud to reinforce its potential in your life.
- As you hold a yoga pose, reflect on the virtues or attitudes associated with that pose. (The poses and their respective attitudes are listed with each of the poses described in this chapter.) Create an affirmation or mantra to cultivate this attitude and program that mental state into your body. Repeat the mantra or affirmation as you hold a yoga pose or move through a series of them.

- Observe how creating the shapes of yoga poses gives you new experiences with your body, offering you fresh ways to relate to yourself. Doing so can open your eyes to the dynamic nature of your body and all its parts. This can be a helpful way to learn how to objectively observe your body versus subjectively judging it.

- Pause in a pose from time to time to engage in self-study by observing your self-talk. Pay attention to how your self-talk, both positive and negative, influences your body image in that exact moment. Also observe how your self-talk affects how you experience your body in the pose. Just as you did in the Learn section, record the relationship between your words and how you feel about yourself to increase your body mindful self-awareness. If you find yourself leaning more toward body mindless self-talk, incorporate one of the other practices from this chapter to help lead you in the body mindful direction.

- Combine a mantra with the rhythm of your breath as you hold a yoga pose. For example, as you inhale, say "I am unique." As you exhale, say "I am unique." Choose words that are meaningful to you and channel your body mindful goals and intention.

Create Body Mindful Rituals
That Harness Your Strengths

You have a wealth of unique talents, skills, and preferences. In addition to the practices in this chapter that we suggested, we strongly encourage you to create a ritual or two that favors your natural disposition. When you channel your energy in a direction that honors your unique temperament and likes, you have a better chance of nurturing a new personal insight or a desired change. This means that if you like singing, sing. If you find peace from meditation, then meditate on your new insights. If you appreciate group discussion for learning, then seek out like-minded friends. Please take charge of this process and develop a personalized ritual that complements your unique preferences and nature.

For individuals who enjoy movement and writing, a personalized ritual might be combining a yoga pose practice with some quiet time afterward for journaling to reflect on your self-talk during the practice or how you experienced your body in the poses.

Goal-oriented folks might benefit from something like this: Sit or stand in your favorite room in your house, somewhere outdoors, or even at your work desk. Take several deep breaths to create a purposeful pause to remember your body mindful intention, and identify three ways you are going to live your intention that day.

For people who prefer a more passive practice, guided meditation may be a valuable ritual to begin. Seek out guided meditation apps or downloads that resonate with your body mindful intention and fill you with a sense of calm and connectedness. After the meditation, you might do some journaling or list some new insights or inspirations that resulted from the quiet time.

There's no one right way to create a daily personalized ritual, and the options are nearly endless. What's most important is that you harness your strengths and engage with elements of your inner life (like your preferences, passions, and talents) to create a ritual that you look forward to doing and that supports you in your body mindful journey.

Daily Practice Is the Key

Give yourself time to explore which practices and rituals (or combinations of them) resonate best for you. Trust us: You have to do a practice more than once for it to make a difference. It takes a daily commitment. Even more important is the attitude you bring to this Love step. Keeping your mind open to new possibilities and experiences will serve you best. We also encourage you to call on close friends, family, and others with whom you can share your experiences, especially if you are the kind of learner who benefits from processing your feelings and ideas out loud. Having accountability with a trusted person in your life can be helpful in following through with your practices, too.

Chapter Summary

1. Love is the third step of the Butera Method of Personal Transformation and focuses on daily yoga practices to integrate body

mindful language into your life and ultimately cultivate an affirming relationship with your body.

2. Yoga is vast in nature and includes an array of physical, mental, and spiritual practices that originated in ancient Indian philosophy.

3. Explore a variety of mental, physical, auditory, and visual yoga practices to determine which ones align with your learning preferences and resonate with your unique qualities.

4. View these yoga practices as a gift (versus a chore), giving you time and space each day to devote to nurturing your body mindful intention—your heartfelt desire for your relationship with your body.

5. Keep a journal handy to record insights and inspirations.

6. Affirmations are like push-ups for your heart.

7. Expand your learning to all the senses. Like water soaking a garden, permit new patterns to reach you through all the senses.

8. Keep your personal practice space as sacred. This includes eliminating distractions such as devices and other things that take you out of a state of focus.

9. Embody new patterns through yoga poses. Align your breath, mind, and physical posture as an expression of wisdom.

10. Keep at your yoga practices daily. If you miss a day, simply begin again. Let go of the expectation to be perfect at these practices. Doing so will remove critical self-talk from the equation.

11. Empower yourself to honor your talents and gifts and create personalized rituals that incorporate your unique abilities and preferences.

12. Applying these life-affirming concepts and practices to different areas of your life will spark a ripple effect of feeling more and more empowered each day.

You now have yoga practices to deepen your inner life and your relationship with your body. In the next and final step of the Butera Method of Personal Transformation (Live), you will learn supportive ways to model and demonstrate body mindfulness in your interactions with others, so that at the same time you are practicing validating yourself, you are helping others do the same for themselves. The changes you make will be far-reaching as a result of your self-aware interactions with yourself and others in your life.

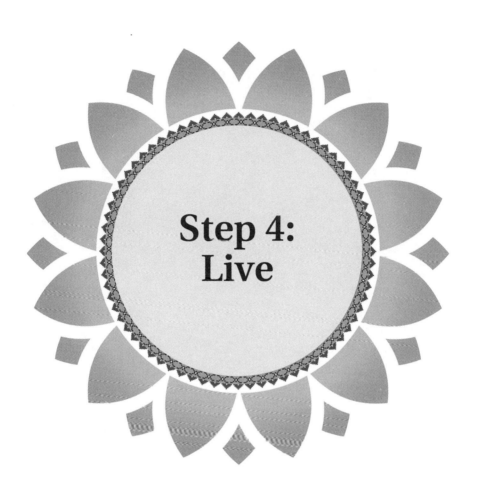

Step 4:
Live

In the Live step, the final step of the Butera Method of Personal Transformation, you will learn strategies for real-life practice in communicating body mindfully during your interactions with others. In the Love step, you learned practices to help you actively integrate the new language you crafted in the Learn step. The Live step is a call to action to consciously choose to model body mindful language for others. Essentially, this means learning how to speak *and* listen to others without the goal of seeking or granting external validation. By using language in this very mindful way with family members, friends, colleagues, and peers and in your personal responses to social messages, you will help others feel more comfortable in their own skin simply by working on this effort within yourself. This is the world that body mindful people can create for one another simply by committing to raising each other up through language that is not dependent on how well our bodies and lives match external values and ideals.

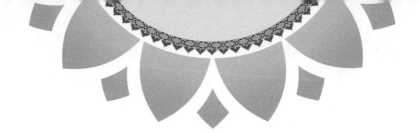

Chapter 12

How to Be a
Body Mindful Ambassador

Welcome to the last step of the Butera Method of Personal Transformation: Live. This step will teach you how to put body mindful into action by living it in the world. To live body mindfully is to be what we call a "body mindful ambassador," because what you practice in yourself will shine through for others. You will naturally manifest and embody empowered, self-validating energy, and your example may even inspire others to make body mindful changes in their own lives. After all, if laughter and happiness are contagious, the same can be true for a positive self-image. This is powerful stuff indeed! The members of our world deserve to feel at ease and validated from within.

The tips outlined in this chapter will support you as you strengthen your own body mindful awareness and create the possibility for family members, friends, colleagues, peers, and others you encounter in your daily life to feel empowered in their bodies and lives because you exude a spirit of acceptance and nonjudgment.

Becoming a Body Mindful Ambassador

Athletes, musical performers, and debate team members are examples of ambassadors. These students represent their school's values and philosophies with pride to their peers, the community, and beyond. You may have memories of behavioral guidelines, dress codes, and tips on how to be a model citizen while at away games or other competitive events. To represent one's school in this way is a privilege.

In the twelve-step Anonymous programs for people dealing with addictions, the final step is mentoring another addicted person into sobriety. Being so strong that you are able to guide another person toward healing demonstrates that you have learned your lessons. Seeing the process work for another human being firsthand teaches you subtle aspects of the twelve-step process that you may not have noticed during your personal self-reflection, proving that there are breakthroughs one can make by watching another.

In the field of martial arts, the expert-level black belt artists maintain their community by teaching the lower-level students. This practice may seem to be a service or an exchange for their own tutelage, but there is another reason for it: it allows the expert to continue to improve. In martial arts there is a belief that when an artist can perform a movement slowly and with correct form, then they have mastered it. In other words, understanding the micro-movements or micro-aspects of a subject can be accomplished by teaching them to others.

These three examples vividly illustrate the Latin proverb *Docendo discimus*: "By teaching, we learn." It's true that teachers do learn by teaching. In fact, many teachers feel they learn more than the students they teach, because the act of educating generates new knowledge to be studied and disseminated.

Believe it or not, you too are now ready to teach. Now that you have developed some positive body mindful insights and habits, those same habits can be taught to others. In the act of teaching, you will learn more and more about your own language, beliefs, and attitudes that influence your body image and self-esteem. As a body mindful ambassador, you will simultaneously teach and learn while paving the way for others to learn and eventually teach through living body mindfully.

The following steps will teach you how to apply the Live step in your daily life. You do not need to apply all of these at once. Since these are new skills, take time practicing them and getting comfortable with them. We recommend that you practice one skill at a time, multiple times, before trying out the next one.

Six Ways to Be a Body Mindful Ambassador

1. Listen to Others with Compassion, Acceptance, and Patience

We predict that cognitive information processing will be a subject of study for all children in the future, not just students with performance issues. Learning style, comprehension abilities, concentration nuances, and the prized skill of listening will all be expertly analyzed. Listening, or the process of comprehending information, impacts every aspect of life, from learning to living to loving. The way you receive information in part alters the information given to you.

The art of listening offers you a window into your information internalization process. Put another way, our internal processing (the thoughts that fire in our own minds as we listen to others speak) is an opportunity to also listen to ourselves. Here's an example: Let's say we included a bunch of politically incorrect or body-shaming words in this book. In that case, not only would this book probably not have made it to print, but you likely would have a running internal dialogue as you read what we had to say. Your internal dialogue would be full of insights about your relationship to those words and how they make you feel. By paying attention to your internal dialogue, you are listening to yourself. Listening to others is for the listener, first and foremost.

Now, let's say you shouted out a body-shaming slur to a police officer. In this situation you could be charged with a crime. But the irony is, if you called yourself a body-shaming name in your mind for no one else to hear, you could get away with it all day long. Listening to this body-shaming name on repeat could lead you to feel depressed, anxious, or maybe even worthless or unlovable.

Here's our very important point: When you practice listening to others with kindness, you train yourself to speak and listen kindly to yourself. Notice we didn't say that when you learn to say nice things to others you will say nice things to yourself. We are all usually pretty good at saying nice things to others. We are talking about *listening* with kindness, not offering praise.

To listen with kindness means you permit others to express their feelings and thoughts and you accept them freely and without question. Acceptance is a gift rarely received or given in our modern day. Few of us are taught to listen with kindness and acceptance. Rather, in Western culture we are taught to speak up, interrupt others, and push our judgments, complaints, advice, and ideas to the forefront.

Here are three ways to listen to others with kindness:

- **Give the other person your full attention.** Don't look at your phone or think about anything extraneous when you're with another person. Gift the other person with your full attention.

- **Be curious.** Don't assume you know what the other person is going to say next. Instead, ask clarifying questions and encourage the person to share what's important to them in that moment.

- **Drop judgment.** This step may take years of practice to master, because in order to be genuine, you must share your opinions and thoughts. However, you may do so while accepting the other person's viewpoint.

When we show genuine interest in another human being, we heal ourselves while healing them. Not only do we practice listening to others, but we also practice listening to ourselves being kind. We show ourselves that kindness comes from within, and with time and practice we can find kindness in our thoughts.

2. Learn from Your Mistakes

First and foremost, know that if you don't always model body mindful language for others and yourself, it's okay. This is a learning process, and it takes time and practice for it to feel more and more natural. We don't expect the ingrained language and beliefs that you may have been carrying for most if not all of your life to simply be dismantled and fall out of existence. We are taught to believe that changing our bodies to match inherited beliefs and social ideals will give us power. We think that if we look and act a certain way that is approved of by others, then we will be able to have friends, a job, a lover, etc. This idea is so instinctive that we freely admit to making mistakes in our own lives. To be honest, both of us are prone to worrying about what we look like while giving lectures, if we are attractive, and whether our students like us, and we wonder if we will truly be able to help our society with the odds stacked against us.

So let's say you make a comment about how so-and-so looks good since they lost some weight. Sure, this statement registers as a compliment in terms of social norms, but although you did not intend to, those words reinforce a detrimental social norm: validation based on weight or dress size. When these small slip-ups occur, note them in your mind and take time to try to understand why they happened. What belief were you propagating at that moment? What pattern did you recreate, and why?

Be gentle with yourself. Notice when you fall into body mindless habits, and make a dedicated effort to reconnect with the body mindful intention you set at the beginning of this book to get you motivated once again. Here is the step-by-step approach we use in our own lives to get back on track:

1. Catch the mistake.
2. Take time to understand it.
3. Reconnect with the original body mindful intention.
4. Begin again on the body mindful path.

Learn from this reflection and then write down a new body mindful comment that validates the other person based on their internal qualities. The more you take this kind approach with others, the more natural it will feel to extend to yourself.

3. Affirm Others for Their Internal Qualities Versus Their External Looks

So many of the polite things we say to others out of habit relate to externals. For example, it is socially acceptable to compliment someone on their clothing. Such a statement could be expressing the opinion that the person looks nice, or it could just be a polite thing to say, even if you don't truly mean it. Either way, the compliment focuses on the person's external appearance.

As another example, "I like your new watch" could be code for "You must be making a lot of money and doing well for yourself" or "You have become a successful adult with lots of money, and money is my measure of your success." Instead of commenting on externals, which in the end only reinforces external validation, you could talk to your friend about what they are doing in their life these days that lights them up. And when you hear (or listen with kindness to) how this friend is doing volunteer work, you might then affirm one of their inner qualities, such as selflessness or generosity. Or you could say to that friend with the shiny watch, "How is work going for you these days?" and get them to talk about how their company helps people with healthcare issues. This kind of conversation allows you to affirm your friend's dedication to improving other people's lives and offers them a much more lasting sense of personal empowerment than an offhand comment about a watch.

Inner qualities you might affirm in others include courage, patience, honesty, diligence, compassion, kindness, dedication, creativity, humor, and lightheartedness. There are many more possibilities, of course, and as you tune in to others' talents and gifts, you will find all kinds of unique words with which to affirm them. Practicing affirming other people's inner qualities is an opportunity to practice this in your own life. Doing so builds personal empowerment and strengthens your resolve, because as you empower others you are simultaneously building yourself up.

4. Do Not "Advice Teach," but Rather "Listen Teach."

People crave direction. Many of us want to be told how to be successful, feel better, lose weight, or overcome challenges. This approach can make the road to happiness easier or be a shortcut, so why wouldn't we pay for some good old advice?

When someone asks you to tell them what to do, to give them marching orders to the land of contentment, the best way to be a body mindful ambassador is to give them a blank map. Instead of giving them advice or talking ad nauseam about yourself, simply ask them how they feel about themselves and then listen with kindness.

They will likely beg you for the keys to happiness. And sometimes you might give in and say, "Do this and then do that. It's what I did, so you should do it too." But instead of taking the bait and spouting off advice (which isn't listening), ask the other person to define the words in the question they asked of you, one at a time.

Here's what we mean. Say someone asks you, "How will I overcome my fear of how my big hips make me unattractive?"

This question is a cultural set-up, as the only answer to this sort of question is to alter your body parts to match an unrealistic external ideal. To be a body mindful ambassador in this situation, try this:

1. Break down the question. Ask the person, "What are 'big hips' to you?" That question may sound crazy, but remember, to be a kind listener is not to assume what the other person means. In truth, you really don't know what they mean by "big hips." You know your definition of this, but you don't know exactly what it means for the other person. You also don't know the belief system or thought process that person values that supports their line of thinking.

    Next, ask what they mean by the word "unattractive." What is the measure of "attractive" for you? For whom are we attractive? Continue to break down every aspect of the person's request for advice.

2. Once you break down their question, you will notice that the questioner will start to rephrase aspects of the original question on their own. Listen to them some more.

3. Ask the person to rephrase the entire question. Yes, after all your questions, ask them how they might rephrase things. You might ask, "So why is it important to you to change your body?" This approach will help the other person get clearer about what it is they want. This step will also help you resist partaking in the cultural assumption that beauty looks a certain way and is only an external entity.

4. Continue to listen to the person and ask questions from a place of curiosity. Doing so will create space for the other person to arrive at the realizations they long to gain about themselves. What is key is your curious attitude. Advice giving will not allow the other person to listen and learn for themselves.

5. Share Your Newfound Joy and Freedom

When your story is of interest to those beyond your immediate family, your sense of self-esteem may swell. It is in these moments that your story may inspire others, especially if you tell it in the first person in a way that does not set you up to rely on other people's impressions and feedback to validate your story.

Just tell your story, and permit the listener to hear whatever they wish. Let them follow in your footsteps if they want to; let them have their own experience. They might latch on to one part of your story, or perhaps your story has no real relevance to them personally but gives them an idea to pursue.

Here are a few quick tips for sharing about yourself with others:

- **Share your beginnings.** Talk freely about yourself, without fear of what others think, as that would be relying on others to validate your experience. Be careful of statements that indicate you are giving advice, such as "In my personal experience..." or "For me...." These statements, although not inherently pushy, can come across as advice giving. Allow yourself to be who you are without qualifying it. Your listeners already know this is your experience, and they can choose to follow your lead if they like.

- **Check in to see if others are still listening.** Keep your story brief, and permit the listener to ask questions if they wish to. Be genuine and honest but not full of yourself. This means that if you are interrupted, you can stop talking and kindly listen without the need to finish. You are telling your story for the listener, not to hear yourself talk. Also, check in with your listener about whether the conversation is helpful. Ask a gentle question like "How are you doing?" and notice their body language. The information you are sharing may be overwhelming to the listener, especially if the person recognizes that their life is driven by external pressures.

- **Share your pain safely and carefully.** If you are sharing intimate fears or problems, even with a friend, be careful how you share this information, as you may make yourself overly vulnerable. In a public setting, be mindful that others might misinterpret your pain as weakness. "I am self-conscious about my body" is a clear statement and maintains your personal boundaries, whereas "I am self-conscious about my body image because as a kid people joked at my expense about my big ears, and I worked for years to deal with this" is a statement that could set you up for people to be your caretaker or maybe even your future bully.

- **Share your insights.** Give life to statements that are inherently true, and explain how they work for you. An example of this is "I choose to look at fitness from the perspective of health, and this shift helped me stop overexercising. It also made me aware that my nutrition and rest are important." Give examples to help others understand things, and keep those examples succinct. Once we become preachy, our language may fall out of line with body mindful in our efforts to convince or even control others.

- **Share how you created new habits.** Insights lead to practice, and over time the practice becomes routine or habit. Explain the journey of how your language shifted using the body mindful approach. Did you take extra courses or practice with friends? Did you journal a lot or do some meditation or yoga? Remember that your habits are an example, not a blueprint. Offer people options so that your habits are not seen as the only choice for growth. Share a story about a friend or someone else inspiring who may have a unique story. Keep all these stories brief.

- **Explain how you are transforming language.** *Body Mindful Yoga* is based on one key principle: being mindful of language versus permitting your language patterns to define you. This means you must craft your words and examine how they are affecting your self-esteem, your compassion, your sense of beauty, and your identity.

As an example, let's say your boss raises her voice at you and your coworkers. You think to yourself, "I am a bad person because my boss yelled at all of us staffers." This thought brings you down and gets you thinking about all the other ways you are a "bad person" in your life.

Instead of turning your boss's words and actions on yourself, you might rewrite that initial thought as "Oh, that is my boss trying to motivate me with fear." This revision has an entirely different vibe, one that allows you to deflect versus absorb your boss's words and not feel bad about yourself. You also allow your boss to be who she is without taking responsibility for her feelings. This, too, is a form of listening with kindness.

As you practice this kind of language shifting for yourself, you will be able to help others by listening with kindness to their reactions and, through asking qualifying questions, guiding them to shift their own reactions and find freedom from disempowering thoughts.

You can also share with others what words, expressions, and slogans are hot buttons for you. Share about the areas in your own life where you are practicing body mindful language. Perhaps it's in how you speak and listen to your spouse or children or to your coworkers or customers.

6. Remain Non-attached or Neutral

Your enthusiasm for living body mindfully may not always be met with the same energy. Heck, you may not always feel sure of yourself as you continue this personal journey. Therefore, it's important to remember that if you want everyone in your life to learn the same lessons you have learned, you will likely be let down, because, as the famous idiom goes, "You can lead a horse to water, but you can't make him drink." Our family and friends (and even ourselves) will only be able to change when they are ready.

Others may negate your ideas by saying things like "Yes, but…" or "Yes, well, I am still going to…" or "Maybe I will try that." It's best for you to expect that they will continue to do what they are doing, even if it pains you to see how they are selling themselves short. When someone resists and you respond by challenging them or pushing back and defending yourself, then you are not being sensitive to the choices they are making. When making the decision to change, a "pros and cons" process must always occur. Our minds were designed to stick with things that work. It makes sense to us to do what we did yesterday. So expect resistance and figure that it is a step on the journey to change.

In the field of psychology, there is a helpful chart that describes the process of change. James Prochaska and Carlo DiClemente outlined these steps in 1983 for smoking cessation.[33] This model of behavioral change explains how altering our behavior is a circuitous journey rather than a straight line to ascend.

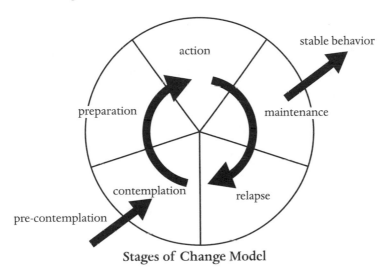

Stages of Change Model

THE STAGES OF CHANGE:

Stage 1: Pre-contemplation

Stage 2: Contemplation

Stage 3: Preparation

Stage 4: Action

Stage 5: Maintenance

Stage 6: Relapse

Stage 7: Stable Behavior

33. James O. Prochaska and Carlo C. DiClemente, "Stages and Processes of Self-Change of Smoking: Toward an Integrative Model of Change," *Journal of Consulting and Clinical Psychology* 51, no. 3 (June 1983): 390–395, doi.org/10.1037/0022-006X.51.3.390.

When a person first hears of *Body Mindful Yoga*, it may appear fascinating to them, but they are merely hearing about the book. They are in the beginning stage of Pre-contemplation. Pushing a person in the beginning is like pushing them away from the goal, because they aren't yet moving. Once they hear about or read *Body Mindful Yoga*, they may move into Contemplation, which is considering the benefits of making a change. If just reading the book is a Contemplation, it could move a person along to the action step, since there are so many exercises in the book. However, if the person is truly ready, then they might prepare to make a change.

Once a person acts, they create true momentum. The thing to remember is that one stressful event or setback can move a person back down the ladder. The biggest challenge arises after a person makes a positive change and maintains it, because inevitably life will arrange a setback. At the point of Relapse, if the person knows upfront to expect a setback, then they can make the relapse shorter in duration and go back into a maintenance phase. The truth is we are all going to have relapses, and one of the qualities of wisdom is to accept your relapse so quickly that no one need suffer.

Where to Go From Here

Continuing with your own body mindful journey is the best possible way to be an ambassador for others. This means keeping up with daily yoga practices and consciously applying body mindful awareness and skills every day to your spoken and unspoken language, your interactions with others, and your responses to social messages. Let's think of these steps as a circle that keeps spiraling up toward the infinite so that the process is not rigid. Let's flow in out of these steps so that eventually our thoughts become less harsh and more empowered.

Remember, what you practice in yourself will shine through for others. You will create space in your life for you to be yourself as you do the same for others. Imagine *that* world! This is the world that body mindful people can create for one another.

One Last Exercise

Before moving on to the conclusion, let's take a moment for one final exercise.

EXERCISE: Your Body Mindful Narrative

Since writing your body narrative way back in chapter 3, you have studied your relationship with your body and the world through the lens of language. You have done hard work, and are wiser for it. You likely have some new language to work with in your yoga practice and are ready to try out new skills for interacting with others in body mindful ways that are attuned with your body mindful goals and intention.

Taking all this wisdom and self-awareness into account, write another body narrative—your *body mindful narrative*. What's the new "story" you wish to tell yourself about your body? What words will you choose to integrate into your self-talk and use to speak back to disempowering thoughts and messages? Who is the body mindful you in your inner and outer lives?

Take your time and let the words flow. May this exercise be a celebration of your learning and wisdom and an affirmation of your body and life.

Chapter Summary

1. The Live step is a call to action to consciously choose to speak *and* listen to others without the goal of seeking or granting external validation.

2. By using language in this very mindful way with family members, friends, colleagues, and peers and in your personal responses to social messages, you will help others feel more comfortable in their own skin simply by working on this effort within yourself.

3. You are a body mindful ambassador simply by affirming people for their internal qualities.

4. Listen with kindness to what others are saying. Explore what others mean by their words and ideas.

5. When listening to another person, keep the focus on them by avoiding giving advice or sharing your thoughts until you have listened to them deeply. Give the gift of listening!

6. Learn from your mistakes by understanding the "why" behind your words and actions. View your mistakes as learning opportunities.

7. Offer the types of follow-up questions that direct the other person to think from the standpoint of internal validation versus external validation.

8. Share your story when others are interested. Share your beginnings and your growth.

9. Change happens in stages, so give people (and yourself) plenty of time to adjust as they are ready.

10. Consciously bring all four steps of the Butera Method of Personal Transformation into your life in your spoken and unspoken language, your interactions with others, and your responses to social messages.

As you continue to model affirming self-talk and language with others, you will continue to improve your own inner resolve. Think of empowering yourself in body mindful ways around others in order to remain humble and respectful, versus thinking that you have to correct others. Let's all commit to improving our awareness of the far-reaching power of our words.

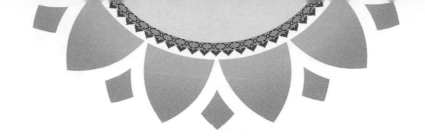

Conclusion:
Beyond Words

Although this is the conclusion of the book, it's hardly the end of your body mindful journey. In many ways you are just getting started! The abundance of new insights that have emerged because of your self-study and new practices are fresh ground from which to shape a self-empowered body image. As a newly minted body mindful ambassador, you have the exciting opportunity to test out new language with yourself and others. We encourage you to approach this process with curiosity and to stay open to trying out words that resonate with your body mindful intention.

Remember to be gentle with yourself as you explore this new territory. As you are aware, we don't wake up one day automatically able to use body-affirming language in our thoughts and words. It takes courage to ride the ebb and flow of emotions we experience when working on ourselves. We urge you to stick with it. Every day of your life, stay diligent in your body mindful practices. Be purposeful with your words and vigilant of your thoughts. Talk back to social messages that pull you down with body mindful words that raise you up and guide you to self-validation. You *can* do this!

Word-Free Spaces

Our words matter immensely, as you well know by now! Yet we would like to close by planting one more seed: There exists a space beyond words. Ironically, this sort of experience is difficult to describe in words! People of all ages enjoy activities that focus their mind by having it operate outside the boundaries of words. Athletes use the common phrase "in the zone" to express a peak consciousness that occurs when the athlete has united all their faculties to find the essence of the sport. Musicians experience this when they *feel* the music; jazz musicians often describe being in a "flow state" when they play. Artists of all kinds lose track of time as they immerse themselves in their craft. Experienced practitioners of yoga asana and meditation may also experience a consciousness that is independent of words. Cooks, bakers, gardeners, photographers, hikers, knitters, writers, and many others describe a similar experience.

It is our hunch that people find much peace when they let go of words for periods of time and merge with their sport, craft, music, etc. Perhaps you have an activity in your life that offers this sort of word-free space. In fact, in this same space you may forget about your body, because your consciousness is on a plane totally void of outside forces and pressure.

Incorporating activities and experiences that lead you into the realm beyond words is also a way to practice body mindfulness. In this way, not only are you empowered by being in the zone (connected to something that you truly love doing and that is just for you), but you also tap into an inner peace and show yourself that it *is* possible to embody purely empowered moments and spans of time. Visit this place daily and come home to your highest, wisest, most liberated self. Savor the realm beyond words.

And when you return, may your words affirm your body and embrace your inner wisdom.

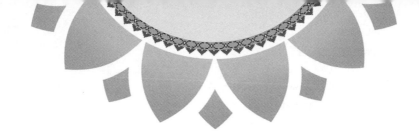

Acknowledgments

From Bob

It is difficult to find the words that express the appropriate amount of gratitude for the many people, places, and things that have contributed to this book coming together. Words seem to fall short, especially when my heart is this full of joy.

First, it has been a pleasure working with my co-author, Jennifer Kreatsoulas. Her enthusiasm for the topic merged with her writing talent to bring this work to life. Jennifer's experiences in teaching yoga to diverse populations initiated the process, and her continued compassion and enthusiasm for the topic ushered the information out into the world in a thoughtful and engaging way.

To all my teachers over the years, your perspectives made my story diverse and your teachings enriched my life in ways that I cannot fully express. To my parents, thank you for encouraging me to travel the world, where I learned that in different places, words and gestures carry varied cultural meanings and significance. In particular, my time studying Chinese, Japanese, and French, along with bits and pieces of many other languages, helped me to see and understand language as an expression of consciousness that shapes our life experiences.

To all of the strong and intelligent women I have learned from and with over the years, thank you. I was very fortunate to have educational experiences that offered a feminist perspective on language that eventually helped me to develop a humanist perspective on language. These learning environments helped me to view the world in new and different ways. I first learned of the more conscious use of language from my prep school classmates at Phillips Academy. This learning continued at the Friends World College, where the Quaker views on equality were embodied in a unique and compelling way. At the Earlham School of Religion, I was fortunate to take classes in which I learned how language has the potential to harm, repress, uplift, or empower different populations. My PhD studies at the California Institute of Integral Studies helped me to integrate Eastern and Western concepts in way that allowed me to teach to a broader audience on a wider variety of subjects. I view this book as an extension of their ongoing mission of diversity and inclusion.

Thank you to my teachers at the Yoga Institute in Mumbai, who taught me yoga as a total lifestyle approach and developed my critical thinking skills with an eye toward compassion and a reverence for all life. I am very lucky that my yoga education included so much breadth and depth. I am still exploring what I learned at the Yoga Institute in a way that continues to compel me to share it with others.

The YogaLife Institute teachers' and support staff's continued commitment to selfless service continually inspires me, and the gifts they bring to the community uplifts us all. It is a joy to call them colleagues and friends. For this project, I was grateful to receive ongoing support from Al Cochrane, Erika Tenenbaum, Jennifer Hilbert, and Kanjana Rajaratnam Hartshorne.

A few people did early read-throughs of the manuscript and offered insightful feedback to improve the execution and delivery of the materials; thank you Jocelyn Moye, Ilene Rosen, Thaine Smith, Devon D'Angelo, Cienna Mattei, and Connie Cullen. More than two hundred people contributed to our initial survey on the topic of body image and honestly addressed several sensitive questions that guided the project.

Thank you to my Yoga Therapy colleagues and students, the International Association of Yoga Therapists, and the team of Comprehensive Yoga Therapy at The YogaLife Institute, for pioneering the field of yoga therapy: Staffan Elgelid, Erin Byron, Larry Payne, Amy Gage, the late Georg Feuerstein, Eleanor Criswell, Dilip Sarcar, John Kepner, and many more.

Thank you to Deby Ross Harrison and to publishing experts Bill and Steve Harrison, who invited us to a Mastermind weekend with bestselling author Jack Canfield that opened up a whole new field of possibility.

Thank you to the team at Llewellyn Worldwide, especially Angela Wix, Andrea Neff, Kat Sanborn, Vanessa Wright Harrison, Molly McGinnis, Larry Kunkel, and Bobbi O'Connor, who all make writing a book far easier and enjoyable than I could have ever imagined!

As always, I am grateful for all the students at the YogaLife Institute, whose depth, sincerity, honesty, and dedication continue to delight and amaze me. In the end, I learn as much, if not more, from them than they do from me. It is their willingness to explore themselves and the depths of yoga that allows me to live my dharma.

I thank my loving wife, Kristen, for following her heart in life and fulfilling our wedding vows of being a "partner on the path of enlightenment." We might have added the line "for better and for book deadlines!" Your unconditional love is a gift from God.

From Jennifer

I am overwhelmed with joy and gratitude for the opportunity to share this book with the world. My mother always told me that my life's experiences would someday serve to help others. Her words planted a seed in my soul that set my life's work in motion. My education, lived experiences, and yoga studies have taught me that the purest way I can help others is to empower them to trust the brilliance of their wisdom. My deepest hope is that our book offers readers a pathway to embody their personal power.

I thank my husband, Constantine, and daughters, Demetra and Zoe, my greatest sources of inspiration. Every day you empower me to live my life to the fullest. My gratitude for your love and support is boundless. I dedicate my life's work to my daughters. May they always know they are loved and safe and that their place and power in this world are not dependent on the size and shape of their bodies.

To my parents, sister, and extended family, thank you for believing in me with a fierceness that could move mountains. To my lifelong best friends, Kristin Mazenko Jakubowski, Jessica Puma Melchiorre, Karen Beyeler, and Lisa Young, thank you for the special gift of history that we share and for all the years of dreaming and laughter that no doubt had a hand in bringing forth this project.

To my co-author, teacher, and mentor, Bob Butera. When we came together to write this book, Bob shared that his intention was to empower me to trust my wisdom and give life to my ideas. He held true to his word, making our collaboration both an incredible learning experience and a time of personal growth. Our mutual respect for each other's gifts and ideas made the countless hours of brainstorming, outlining, discussing, and writing truly fulfilling. Thank you, Bob, for all you have taught me and continue to teach me.

Thank you, Melanie Klein, for writing the foreword to our book. Your remarkable work has opened the door for unprecedented dialogue and action in the field of body image. Thank you for your influence on me and the millions of others who have benefited from your books and the mission of the Yoga and Body Image Coalition. I also thank my community partners in the Coalition for their dedication to empowering all bodies.

Thank you to all my professors at Lafayette College and Lehigh University. My undergraduate and PhD studies in English literature opened my eyes to the potent power of language and critical thinking. My educational experiences at both institutions fostered my passion for writing and taught me to value language as a means of personal empowerment.

Thank you to all my past and present yoga teachers and the Philadelphia-area yoga community. Through yoga you have taught me how to nurture myself and others with compassion. I especially thank my Comprehensive Yoga Therapy teachers who have endowed me with a tremendous educational experience and enlightened me to my purpose, my dharma. Bob Butera, Kristen Butera, Erin Byron, Staffan Elgelid, Erika Tenenbaum, Libby Piper, and Jennifer Hilbert—your brilliance astounds me time and time again.

Thank you to my Yoga Therapy clients, past, present, and future, and my Yoga Therapy colleagues at the YogaLife Institute for all you have taught me by your example of curiosity, generosity, and courage. I am in awe. Special thanks to Kanjana Rajaratnam Hartshorne, my friend and Yoga Therapy colleague, for your bright mind and heart.

I thank the women who have modeled empowerment in its highest form by holding space for my healing: Linda Hershman, Lindsay Breeden, Elise Tropea, Beth Rosenbaum, Natalie Loschiavo, Kristin Gore, Karen Forbes, Colleen Baratka, Alpa Bhatt, and Beth Knudson.

To the eating disorder community throughout the world, thank you for the profound connection we share. I especially thank my "TSAB family" at the Renfrew Center in Radnor, PA, and the Renfrew community at large, which gave me a solid foundation from which to thrive. I also thank Emily Dumas and my colleagues at Monte Nido Philadelphia, all of whom never miss an opportunity to express their appreciation of Yoga Therapy for their clients.

Special thanks to all who read through the manuscript and offered helpful feedback and editorial support, particularly Colleen Clemens, Heather Flyte, and Tzivya Green. I also thank the two hundred people who kindly took our survey and inspired much of the content for this book.

To the team at Llewellyn Worldwide, especially Angela Wix, Andrea Neff, Kat Sanborn, Vanessa Wright Harrison, Molly McGinnis, Larry Kunkel, and Bobbi O'Connor, thank you for your hard work and kind guidance throughout the writing and publishing process.

Finally, I thank all the children in my life—Demetra, Zoe, Troy, Alexander, Destiny, Anthony, and Michael—who continually enlighten me to what it means to be free and at ease in one's body. May you always embrace peace of body and mind.

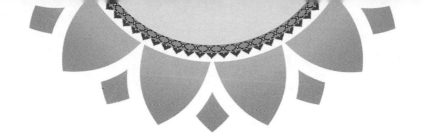

Index

To Write to the Authors

If you wish to contact the authors or would like more information about this book, please write to the authors in care of Llewellyn Worldwide Ltd. and we will forward your request. Both the authors and the publisher appreciate hearing from you and learning of your enjoyment of this book and how it has helped you. Llewellyn Worldwide Ltd. cannot guarantee that every letter written to the authors can be answered, but all will be forwarded. Please write to:

Robert Butera, PhD, and Jennifer Kreatsoulas, PhD
℅ Llewellyn Worldwide
2143 Wooddale Drive
Woodbury, MN 55125-2989

Please enclose a self-addressed stamped envelope for reply,
or $1.00 to cover costs. If outside the U.S.A., enclose
an international postal reply coupon.

Many of Llewellyn's authors have websites with additional information and resources. For more information, please visit our website at http://www.llewellyn.com.

GET MORE AT LLEWELLYN.COM

Visit us online to browse hundreds of our books and decks, plus sign up to receive our e-newsletters and exclusive online offers.

- **Free tarot readings • Spell-a-Day • Moon phases**
- **Recipes, spells, and tips • Blogs • Encyclopedia**
- **Author interviews, articles, and upcoming events**

GET SOCIAL WITH LLEWELLYN

Find us on 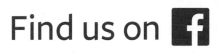 🐦 **@LlewellynBooks**

www.Facebook.com/LlewellynBooks

GET BOOKS AT LLEWELLYN

LLEWELLYN ORDERING INFORMATION

 Order online: Visit our website at www.llewellyn.com to select your books and place an order on our secure server.

 Order by phone:
- Call toll free within the US at 1-877-NEW-WRLD (1-877-639-9753)
- We accept VISA, MasterCard, American Express, and Discover.
- Canadian customers must use credit cards.

✉ **Order by mail:**
Send the full price of your order (MN residents add 6.875% sales tax) in US funds plus postage and handling to: Llewellyn Worldwide, 2143 Wooddale Drive, Woodbury, MN 55125-2989

POSTAGE AND HANDLING

STANDARD (US):
(Please allow 12 business days)
$30.00 and under, add $6.00.
$30.01 and over, FREE SHIPPING.

INTERNATIONAL ORDERS,
INCLUDING CANADA:
$16.00 for one book, plus $3.00 for each additional book.

Visit us online for more shipping options. Prices subject to change.

FREE CATALOG!

To order, call
1-877-
NEW-WRLD
ext. 8236
or visit our
website

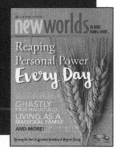

"*Yoga and Body Image* reminds us that it's not what we look like, but how
we live that is the measure of our yoga practice." –Cyndi Lee, author of *May I Be Happy*

MELANIE KLEIN & ANNA GUEST-JELLEY

Including Alanis Morissette,
Seane Corn, Bryan Kest,
Rolf Gates, Dr. Sara Gottfried,
and Linda Sparrowe

YOGA

25 Personal Stories

About Beauty, Bravery

& Loving Your Body

AND BODY IMAGE

Yoga and Body Image
25 Personal Stories About Beauty, Bravery & Loving Your Body
MELANIE KLEIN AND ANNA GUEST-JELLEY

In this incredible, first-of-its-kind book, twenty-five authors, including Alanis Morissette, Seane Corn, Bryan Kest, and Dr. Sara Gottfried, discuss how yoga and body image intersect. With these inspiring personal stories, learn how yoga not only affects your body but also how it affects the way you feel about your body.

Each author offers a unique perspective on how yoga has shaped his or her life and provides tips for using yoga to find self-empowerment and a renewed body image. By bringing together a diverse collection of voices that span the spectrum of human experience, this anthology will help you learn to love your body and embrace a healthy lifestyle.

978-0-7387-3982-3, 288 pp., 6 x 9 **$17.99**

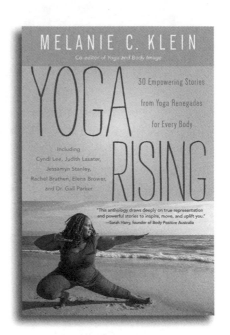

MELANIE C. KLEIN

Co-editor of Yoga and Body Image

YOGA

30 Empowering Stories

from Yoga Renegades

for Every Body

Including
Cyndi Lee, Judith Lasater,
Jessamyn Stanley,
Rachel Brathen, Elena Brower,
and Dr. Gail Parker

RISING

"This anthology draws deeply on true representation
and powerful stories to inspire, move, and uplift you."
—Sarah Harry, founder of Body Positive Australia

Yoga Rising
30 Empowering Stories from Yoga Renegades for Every Body
Melanie C. Klein

Yoga Rising is a collection of personal essays meant to support your journey toward self-acceptance and self-love. This follow-up to the groundbreaking book *Yoga and Body Image* features thirty contributors who share stories of major turning points. Explore how body image and yoga intersect with race and ethnicity, sexual orientation, gender identity, dis/ability, socioeconomic status, age, and size as part and parcel of culture and society.

Collectively, we can make space for yoga that is body positive and accessible to the full range of human diversity. With a special emphasis on how you can take action to build community and challenge destructive attitudes and structures, *Yoga Rising* is a resource for the continuing work of healing ourselves and our world as we move toward liberation for all.

978-0-7387-5082-8, 336 pp., 6 x 9   **$17.99**

To order, call 1-877-NEW-WRLD or visit llewellyn.com
Prices subject to change without notice

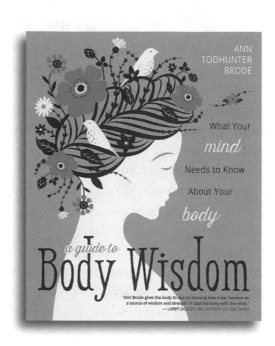

ANN
TODHUNTER
BRODE

What Your
mind
Needs to Know
About Your
body

a guide to
Body Wisdom

"Ann Brode gives the body its due by showing how it can function as
a source of wisdom and strength in total harmony with the mind."
— LARRY DOSSEY, MD, AUTHOR OF *ONE MIND*

A Guide to Body Wisdom
What Your Mind Needs to Know About Your Body
Ann Todhunter Brode

Deepen your spirituality, heal old wounds, and enhance your emotional and physical wellness by engaging in a conversation with your body. This innovative, down-to-earth guide teaches you how to listen to, understand, and work with your body's innate wisdom in everyday living.

A Guide to Body Wisdom provides step-by-step instruction on how to create a personalized self-care regimen that works. You'll learn to quiet your mind and live consciously in your body through a variety of practices, including breathwork, mindful eating, meditation, affirmation, and positive habit building. Featuring simple exercises and techniques, as well as a Body IQ quiz, this valuable book helps you end negative thinking, develop intuition, improve relationships, boost creativity and personal power, and much more.

978-0-7387-5695-0, 288 pp., 7 ½ x 9 ¼　　　　　　　**$21.99**

Praise for *Body Mindful Yoga*

"A wonderful workbook that will lead anyone who has struggled with body image on a journey to healing and self-compassion. A must-read!"
—Melainie Rogers, MS, RDN, CDN, CEDRD-S, founder and CEO
of BALANCE Eating Disorder Treatment Center

"This eminently practical book conveys advice for the cultivation of one's innate power, knowledge, dignity, and capacity to help others. It gives tips for countering competitiveness and the influences of social media. Through yoga and mindful awareness as taught in this book, one discovers how to develop a positive body image and healthy outlook."
—Christopher Key Chapple, Director of the Master of Arts in Yoga
Studies and Doshi Professor of Indic and Comparative Theology
at Loyola Marymount University

"*Body Mindful Yoga* is an excellent tool in the journey of getting to know yourself. Yoga is the art and science of self-study, and this book helps along the path to greater self-awareness. Peace within can only foster peace without."
—Dianne Bondy, E-RYT 500, creator of Yoga For All online training

"From challenging social media 'thinspiration,' 'bikini bodies,' and 'yoga selfies' to creating food neutrality, internal validation, and your own body mindful slogans, this book is full of empowerment. I would highly recommend it to anyone recovering from body hatred, as well as those wanting to cultivate a mindful, compassionate, and empowered relationship with their body."
—Dr. Linda Shanti McCabe, PsyD, author of *The Recovery Mama*
Guide to Maintaining Your Eating Disorder Recovery
in Pregnancy and Postpartum

"This book provides wellness committees, wellness coaches, and executives more tools to support the culture of employee wellness."
—Patricia A. Sullivan, PhD, Leadership and Wellness Coach

"*Body Mindful Yoga* reminds us that the words we choose not only reflect our underlying attitudes towards others and ourselves but also carry a lot of force and resonance that can alter our experience of life either toward or away from balance. Like many forces in nature, our thought patterns can develop momentum and inertia....This book is a valuable source of insight, knowledge, and tools to reform your experience of life."
—Brian Serven, C-IAYT, E-RYT 500, YACEP

"*Body Mindful Yoga* is a bridge to uproot the linguistic and physical injustices of systemic and historical oppression by helping readers forge a pathway to their true and authentic selves—a guidebook and roadmap to reclaim our body narratives. As someone fully recovered from a decade-long eating disorder, yoga was instrumental to my healing. I wish I had had this book when I was in my darkest days."
—Caroline Rothstein, writer, performer, and educator

"Butera and Kreatsoulas have created something truly special: a catalyst for any person ready to reclaim their body image story and finally transform their relationship with their body. Contained within these pages are essential inquiries into your own narrative, and the next steps toward collective liberation. This is quickly becoming my go-to recommendation."
—Jenny Copeland, PsyD, yoga teacher and licensed psychologist at the Ozark Center

"Kreatsoulas and Butera help us see the universe of language that exists within each of us, and how the ways in which we speak silently but continuously to ourselves create our unique body-related thoughts, feelings, and behaviors. By looking more deeply at the words we use internally and externally and offering thoughtful contemplations, they guide us to transform our self-talk to be compassionate, nurturing, and ultimately loving."
—Jenna Hollenstein, MS, RDN, author of *Eat to Love*